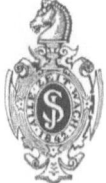

Recent Results in Cancer Research

Fortschritte der Krebsforschung

Progrès dans les recherches sur le cancer

29

Springer-Verlag Berlin Heidelberg GmbH 1970

Aseptic Environments and Cancer Treatment

Edited by

Georges Mathé

With 19 Figures

Springer-Verlag Berlin Heidelberg GmbH 1970

Proceedings of the plenary session of the European Organization for Research on Treatment of Cancer (E.O.R.T.C.) and its cooperative groups. Paris, June 1969

GEORGES MATHÉ, Professeur de Cancérologie Experimentale à la Faculté de Médecine de Paris. Directeur de l'Institut de Cancérologie et d'Immunogénétique, Hôpital Paul-Brousse, F-94 Villejuif

Sponsored by the Swiss League against Cancer

ISBN 978-3-662-30500-3   ISBN 978-3-662-30498-3 (eBook)
DOI 10.1007/978-3-662-30498-3

Recent Results in Cancer Research

Fortschritte der Krebsforschung

Progrès dans les recherches sur le cancer

29

Edited by

Springer-Verlag Berlin Heidelberg GmbH 1970

Aseptic Environments and Cancer Treatment

Edited by

Georges Mathé

With 19 Figures

Springer-Verlag Berlin Heidelberg GmbH 1970

Proceedings of the plenary session of the European Organization for Research on Treatment of Cancer (E.O.R.T.C.) and its cooperative groups. Paris, June 1969

GEORGES MATHÉ, Professeur de Cancérologie Experimentale à la Faculté de Médecine de Paris. Directeur de l'Institut de Cancérologie et d'Immunogénétique, Hôpital Paul-Brousse, F-94 Villejuif

Sponsored by the Swiss League against Cancer

ISBN 978-3-662-30500-3   ISBN 978-3-662-30498-3 (eBook)
DOI 10.1007/978-3-662-30498-3

Preface

The 1969 Proceedings of the Plenary Session of the European Organization for Research on Treatment of Cancer have been divided between two volumes of a completely different nature.

Volume 29, Aseptic Environments and Cancer Treatment, deals not only with the treatment of all types of cancer but also with aplastic treatment of bone marrow and certain other pathological conditions, such as immunological insufficiency, burns etc. Hence the volume will be of interest not only to carcinologists and haematologists but also to paediatricians, surgical units, intensive-care units, hospital administrators and architects and engineers who specialize in hospital design and equipment.

Volume 30, Advances in the Treatment of Acute (Blastic) Leukemias, deals with a particular form of cancer and will have a more restricted readership of carcinologists specializing in leukemia and all haematologists.

Paris, April 1970   GEORGES MATHÉ

Contents

The Aseptic Unit Essential to a Modern Hospital

Introduction

Georges Mathé

Human beings share their environment with a great variety of other living things, the micro-organisms being one of them. Man is in constant contact with bacteria and viruses, and carries a variety of these micro-organisms, the natural defences of the body being protection against their harmful effects. Under certain conditions man can carry pathogenic organisms without ill effects to himself. The micro-organisms which can live quite harmlessly when carried by normal subjects can become dangerous if the host is debilitated, especially if his illness is accompanied by a lack of granulocytes, or insufficiency of immunological reactions.

It is known that man frequently carries pathogenic organisms in the nose, pharynx, around the anus and under the nails, and their circulation between these sites maintains a vicious circle of infection in the carrier. This circle can be broken easily by local applications of antiseptics and antibiotics.

More than 30 per cent of doctors and nurses working in general hospitals are carriers of pathogenic organisms. This percentage can be much higher in oncological or haematological wards, which become reservoirs of pathogens, due to the many patients with myeloid aplasia or infected patients who are nursed in these wards. Attention has been drawn to this scandalous state of affairs—it has been shown that patients died of infections with micro-organisms picked up whilst in hospital.

Under the present, ineffective organisation of hospitals, the susceptible patient cannot be protected from hospital infection except by keeping him as an outpatient, which is only suitable for patients in good general condition, or by nursing in a pathogen-free unit.

In 1956, when we made our first trials of bone marrow grafts in leukaemic patients prepared by total body irradiation [1], we devised a prototype pathogen free unit with the resources available at that time. In 1958, we treated six persons who were accidentally irradiated in Jugoslavia [2], and took advantage of the public interest in the treatment to raise funds to set up far more efficient pathogen-free rooms.

In 1964, when the Institute of Cancerology and Immunogenetics was built at Paul Brousse Hospital, we were able to construct a specially designed unit [3]. The unit, of five "pathogen-free" rooms, has been in use for the past five years and has proved to be of immense practical importance [4]. Patients without circulating granulocytes or immunological defences have stayed in these rooms for several months with no signs of infection.

It would be easy, but scientifically dishonest, to demonstrate the efficiency of our pathogen-free isolation unit by comparing the frequency of infection in patients with the same degree of cytopenia, nursed in this unit, to those nursed in our conventional ward. However, the patients and staff are carefully controlled by weekly bacteriological examination of swabs from the nose, throat, nails and anus; only those having negative results are allowed to enter the pathogen-free rooms. This means that the staff and patients are a selected population; hence, it is true that these pathogen-free units are available for only a limited number of patients, i. e. those who do not carry pathogenic organisms and those in whom the pathogens can be eradicated.

This means that, although the pathogen-free isolation units are useful and are a fundamental requirement, they are not the solution to the problem of hospital infection. We have described the concept of a series of wards in which there is a gradient of microbiological environment, which may offer a solution to this serious problem—the pathogen-free unit is only part of the system.

Since we have used the isolation unit, several European and American groups have used, and improved on, this system. Experience of using these units is published in their report to the annual plenary meeting of the O.E.R.T.C. and includes two interesting topics: the medical application of an aseptic environment, particularly in cancer therapy, and the technology of how the different types of installation can be built to-day. It is hoped that this report will make medical opinion aware of the deplorable conditions existing at present.

Hospitals are badly designed for their primary purpose and, for some patients, are a trap rather than a refuge. Whatever their apparent luxury, their architectural originality or the refinement of their automated administration, they still remain what they were fifty years ago—more infected and more infectious than the street and the underground train.

It is time to build hospitals and wards not just to have beds in them, but to cure patients.

References

1. Mathé, G.: Transfusion et greffe de cellules myéloïdes chez l'Homme. In: Colloque International sur les Problèmes biologiques des Greffes. Liège 18—21 Mars 1959, Université de Liège, ed.
2. — Jammet, H., Pendic, B., Schwarzenberg, L., Duplan, J. F., Maupin B., Latarjet, R., Larrieu, M. J., Kalic, D., Djukic, Z.: Transfusions et greffes de moelle osseuse homologue chez des humains irradiés à haute dose accidentellement. Rev. franç. Étud. clin. biol. 4, 226 (1959).
3. — Forestier, P.: Un outil moderne de la recherche médicale française de l'Institut de Cancérologie et d'Immunogénétique. Intrication de la recherche expérimentale et clinique. Conditionnement hyposeptique des animaux et des malades. Techn. hosp. 20, 47 (1965).
4. Schneider, M., Mathé, G., Schwarzenberg, L., Amiel, J. L., Cattan, A., Schlumberger, J. R., Hayat, M., de Vassal, F., Jasmin, Cl., Rosenfeld, Cl.: Three years experience of the clinical use of a pathogen-free isolation unit. Brit. med. J. 1, 836 (1969).

Five Years Experience of the Clinical Use of a Pathogen-Free Isolation Unit

G. Mathé, M. Schneider, L. Schwarzenberg, J. L. Amiel, A. Cattan,
J. R. Schlumberger, M. Hayat, F. de Vassal, Cl. Jasmin, and Cl. Rosenfeld

Institut de Cancérologie et d'Immunogénétique, Hôpital Paul-Brousse 14,
Avenue Paul-Vaillant-Couturier, 94-Villejuif, France

With 3 Figures

Intensive chemotherapy and radiotherapy in current use in the treatment of malignant disease have given some outstanding results (Mathé et al., 1968) but they can cause, virtually inevitably, periods of profound hypo- or aplasia of the haemopoietic and lymphopoietic systems, whose main complication is infection. Infection has become one of the principal problems in the practice of modern cancer therapy, being particularly formidable in malignant disease of the haemopoietic system, especially in leukaemic, where bone marrow insufficiency is often present before giving any treatment. In a recent study of acute leukaemia, treated with intensive chemotherapy, Frei and his colleagues (1965) reported 60 per cent incidents of bacterial infection with 40 per cent of septicaemia, and 64 per cent incidents of fungal infections with 34 per cent of septicaemia. Autopsy examination has confirmed that infection is the commonest direct cause of death in these cases.

To obtain further progress in the treatment of cancer and especially in treatment of malignancy of the haemopoietic system, it is necessary to reduce the risk of the patient becoming infected. It is with this objective in mind that we have set up, in the Institut de Cancérologie et d'Immunogénétique (Hôpital Paul-Brousse), a pathogen-free isolation unit (P.F.I.U.) (Mathé and Forestier, 1965; Schneider et al., 1969).

In this paper we describe the experience gained from this unit in clinical practice for five years.

I. Material and Methods

1. The Design of the Unit

Fig. 1 shows that this P.F.I.U. comprises, first of all, a series of ante-rooms which ensure that personnel and materials can only gain access into the sterile "sections" after rigorous precautions: a) for personnel, there is a non-sterile changing room,

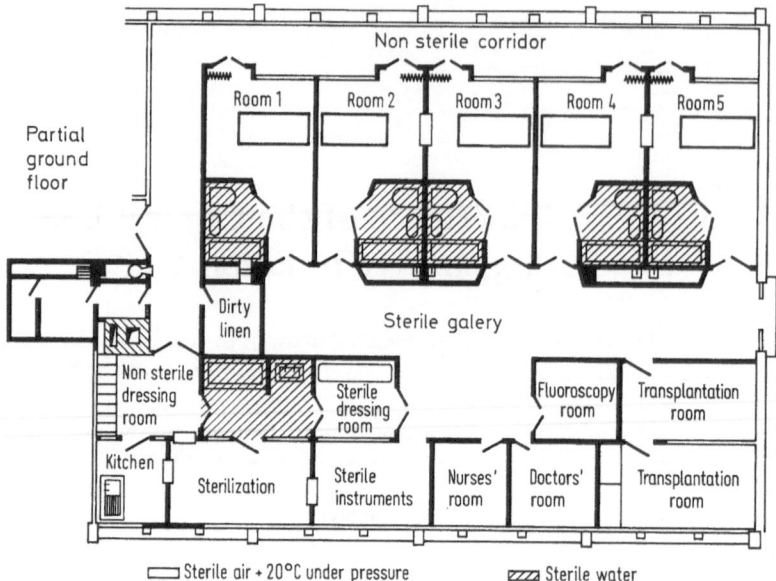

Fig. 1. Plan of the pathogen-free isolation unit at the Institut de Cancérologie et d'Immuno-génétique

a disinfection room and a sterile changing room; b) for materials there is a ster-ilising room, autoclave, and a sterile storeroom; the suite is made up of several rooms, operating theatre, X-ray diagnosis room, rooms for the medical and nursing staff, and five rooms for the patients (Fig. 2). These rooms open through an air-lock onto the internal corridor of the P.F.I.U., they also open via another air-lock, onto a non-sterile corridor. This non-sterile corridor is irradiated for twelve hours a day by five ultra-violet lamps. If a patient becomes infected, he can either be excluded from the sterile suite or be looked after via the non-sterile corridor after his room had been isolated from the remainder of the sterile unit. The patient's family can see him from the non-sterile corridor and can talk to him by using an inter-phone.

The incoming air is first drawn through two series of filters and then sterilised by passing it through a tunnel in which twelve large, U.V. lamps are arranged in a circular fashion; it is then humidified with atomised, sterile water and pumped into the P.F.I.U. under positive preasure, at a constant temperature of 20° C. The U.V. lamps are installed in all the rooms of the P.F.I.U. and are lit at least 12 hours a day. An apparatus to produce an aerosol of hexyl resorcinol [1] (MACKAY, 1952) giving an air concentration of 0.1 mgs per cubic metre is used in each room system-atically for 3 hours per day. Water is sterilised by U.V. light. Waste water is not poured directly into the general drainage system of the building, so as to avoid the risk of any infection ascending from the sewers; the water is collected into containers which are removed, along with any other soiled material, from the air-lock leading onto the non-sterile corridor. Materials and food that are being brought into the P.F.I.U. are steam sterilised.

----

[1] AEROVAP

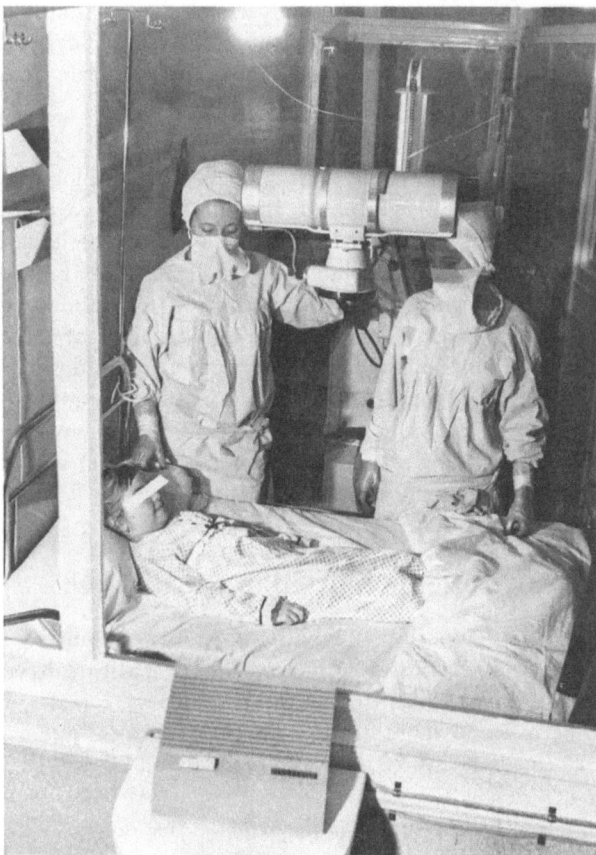

Fig. 2. Photograph of the exterior of a pathogen-free room at the Institut de Cancérologie
et d'Immunogénétique

2. Bacteriological Control of the Personnel and the Isolation Unit

Each week the medical and nursing staff, and members of the family authorised
to enter into the Isolation Unit, undergo a bacteriological investigation, in which
samples are taken from the nose, throat, the ears, the skin, the urine, the faeces and
anus. These specimens are examined for the pathogenic bacteria, pathogenic fungi or
a heavy growth of a single strain of an organism that is to be commonplace. If the
person is carrying one of these categories of organisms, he is temporarily excluded
from the Isolation Unit and treated until this organism disappears. Each week, the
air of the P.F.I.U. is analysed after taking a sample by the sedimentation technique,
using Petri dishes containing trypticase soya gelatine, or Chapman's medium, or
Sabouraud's medium. Swabs taken from various materials are examined for the
presence of organisms. If a pathogen is discovered in one of the rooms, this is then
shut and the walls cleaned with bleaching liquid (eau de javel), the ultra-violet
lights are switched on for 48 hours continuously, and the Hexyl resorcinol atomiser
run continuously for the same time.

Staff entering the P.F.I.U. first take off their clothes in the non-sterile changing room, wash their hands and forearms in an antiseptic bactericidal solution (Phisohex) for five minutes, and then put on sterile clothing in the sterile changing room.

3. Bacterial Control of the Patients

The patients are submitted to the same intensive bacteriological investigation as the personnel before entering the P.F.I.U., and this is repeated twice a week during they stay in the Unit. Only patients in whom no pathogens have been discovered are allowed to enter the Unit. During their stay, they do not receive any pro-phylactic antibiotic treatment, with the exception of mouthwashes containing Nystatine several times a day. When there are clinical signs of infection, antibiotics are only used after the results of the bacteriological examinations have been received, except when the clinical signs indicate there is a very severe infection. In that case, a combination of drugs are given having a very large antibacterial spectrum (Cephalosporine + gentamycine or methicilline + kanamycine) which is later changed according to the results of the sensitivity tests.

II. Patients Nursed in the P.F.I.U.

Over a period of 30 months, 120 patients have been nursed in the P.F.I.U., which is made up of 130 admissions to the Unit (8 patients have been admitted twice, and one three times). Sixty-six of the patients were males, and 54 females; their ages varied between 30 months and 79 years. The total number of days in the Unit has been 3320 (median stay 20 days, the limits 4 and 90 days).

Table 1. *Patients nursed in the pathogen free isolation unit*

Disease	Number of patients	Number of admissions	Reason for admission to the P.F.I.U.	
			Preventive (before chemotherapy)	Neutropenia after chemotherapy
Acute leukaemia	51	60	53	7
Chronic lymphocytic l.	1	1	—	1
Lymphoblastosarcoma	8	8	4	4
Hodgkin's disease	26	26	15	11
Reticulosarcoma	8	8	3	5
Myeloma	1	1	1	—
Polycythaemia	1	1	—	1
Breast cancer	12	12	5	7
Testicular tumours	3	4	4	—
Malignant melanoma	1	1	1	—
Gastro-intestinal tumours	6	6	5	1
Metastasis from a solid undetected primary tumours	1	1	—	1
Bone marrow aplasia (chloramphenicol)	1	1	—	1
Total	120	130	91	39

Table 1 shows the different types of illnesses that were nursed in the Unit. The patients were admitted into the Unit on the basis of two criteria: 1. before giving a form of chemotherapy that was known to cause a very severe neutropenia, or in patients who were neutropenic before the start of treatment; 2. after a previous chemotherapy had caused neutropenia. In each of the 130 courses of treatment, the polymorphonuclear count was or came below 1000/mm^3, and in 95 cases (73 p. cent of the patients) it was less than 500/mm^3.

III. Results

1. Psychological Reactions to the Isolation

We have not observed any severe psychological disturbance in the 120 patients who have been admitted to the Unit. The majority of them were apprehensive about their admission to the P.F.I.U., but tolerated their stay in the Unit perfectly well; this was also true of those patients who remained in the Unit for longer than a month.

2. Infectious Complications

a) General Schedule

Table 2 indicates the types of clinical infections that have been recorded. In the 120 admissions, urinary infections and septicaemia were the most frequent. In 4 cases of septicaemia, the infection was the immediate cause of death.

Table 2. *Types of infections encountered*

Urinary infections	24
Septicaemia	8
Rhinopharyngeal infections	3
Stomatitis	4
Pulmonary infections	1
	40

There is a close relation between the frequency of infection and the number of circulating polymorphonuclear leucocytes, as is shown in Table 3. The total of 1179 days (or 35 per cent of the total) was made up patients who had polymorphonuclear leucocyte counts of less than 500/mm^3, and 31 of the 40 cases of infection (or 77.5 per cent of the total) occured in patients whose granulocytes were less than 500/mm^3. The main bacteria that were found during these infections are shown in Table 4: broadly speaking, they can be considered as enterobacteria (17 cases), pseudomonas (2 cases), streptococci (10 cases), staphylococci (6 cases), alcaligenes (one case). Four infections were observed to be due to Candida albicans, these were predominantly a stomatitis. Finally, routine systematic examination of 11 patients showed the presence of pathogens in the rhinopharynx in 6 cases and in the urine in 5.

Table 3. *The relation between the frequency of infections and the polymorphonuclear leucocyte counts*

Number of infections	Polymorphonuclears/mm³	
	<500	>500
40	31	9

Table 4. *Organisms isolated*

Infections		Carriers discovered during the course of their admission	
E. coli	9		
E. freundii	2		
Klebs. pneumoniae	4		
Proteus vulgaris	1	Proteus vulgaris	2
Proteus mirabilis	1	E. coli	2
Pseud. aeruginosa	2	Staphyloc. aureus	5
Faecalis alcaligenes	1	Klebs. pneumoniae	1
Staphyloc. aureus	6	Pseud. aeruginosa	1
Streptoc. faecalis	10		
Candida albicans	4		

b) Analysis of the Results

α) In Acute Leukaemia (Table 5)

In 61 cases of acute leukaemia, we have seen 15 mild infections, 3 severe infections that were controlled by treatment, and 4 lethal infections (septicaemia), these last 7 cases were in a very advanced state of their disease when the chemotherapy had been undertaken after admitting them to the P.F.I.U. These infections were found when intensive chemotherapy had been used to treat patients in an detectable phase of their leukaemia, associated with severe bone marrow insufficiency, and after they had been submitted to multiple chemotherapy.

β) In Lymphoma

Table 6 indicates that, whatever was the indication for admitting the patient to the P.F.I.U., and despite the frequency of neutropenia, no severe infection was observed in 43 admissions.

γ) In Solid Tumours

Infections were rare, only one severe infection was observed in 24 admissions (Table 7).

δ) One patient was admitted to the Unit having presented with myeloid aplasia following treatment with chloramphenicol. She was hospitalised in the P.F.I.U. for 83 days; for the first 54 days, the level of the polymorphonuclear leucocytes count was less than 500 per mm³, as shown in Fig. 3. She was given no treatment with antibiotics and during this time was afebrile and no infection occured.

Table 5. *Neutropenia and its associated infections in acute leukaemic patients*

Reason for admission	Number for admissions	Polymorphonuclear leucocytes/mm³			Total duration of stay in P.F.I.U.	Body temperature above 38° C		Number of patients with infections		
		<500		>500						
		Number of patients	Number of days	Number of days		Number of patients	Number of days	Mild	Severe	Lethal
Preventive	53	47	689	986	1675	27	178	13 [a]	3	4
Post chemotherapy	8	7	33	87	120	1	4	0	0	0

[a] Two of these patients had two infections.

Table 6. *Neutropenia and its associated infections in patients with lymphoma*

Reason for admission	Number of admissions	Polymorphonuclear leucocytes/mm³			Total duration of stay in P.F.I.U.	Body temperature above 38° C		Number of patients with infections		
		<500		>500						
		Number of patients	Number of days	Number of days		Number of patients	Number of days	Mild	Severe	Lethal
Preventive	21	13	115	366	481	8	56	5	0	0
Post chemotherapy	22	17	193	282	475	10	55	6 [a]	0	0

[a] One of whom had two infections.

Table 7. *Neutropenia and its associated infections in patients with solid tumours*

Reason for admission	Number of admissions	Polymorphonuclear leucocytes/mm³		
		<500		>500
		Number of patients	Number of days	Number of days
Preventive	15	4	19	338
Post chemotherapy	9	7	76	53

Reason for admission	Total duration of stay in P.F.I.U.	Body temperature above 38° C		Number of patients with infections		
		Number of Patients	Number of days	Mild	Severe	Lethal
Preventive	357	3	13	1	1	0
Post chemotherapy	129	4	33	3 a	0	0

a One of these patients had two infections.

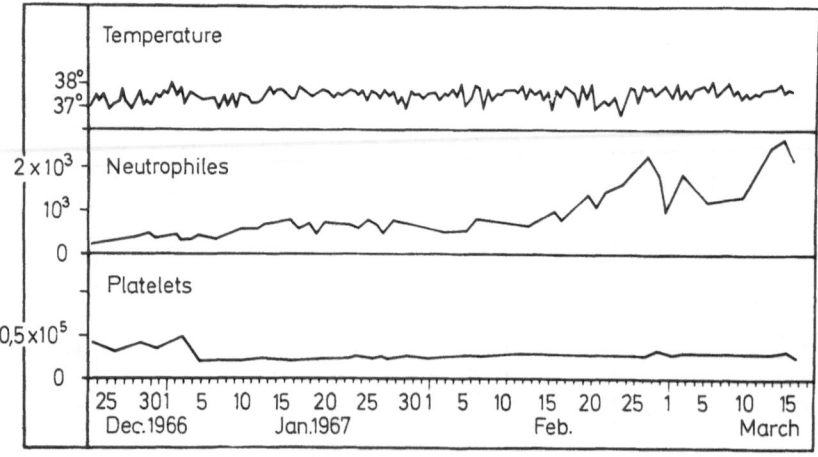

Fig. 3. Temperature chart, neutrophil and platelet counts of a patient who was nursed in a pathogen-free room for 12 weeks and who was not infected although she had a severe neutropenia and thrombocytopenia

In summary, out of 130 courses of treatment in the P.F.I.U., we have counted 32 mild infections, 8 severe infections, of which 4 were lethal; hence, 31 per cent of the patients were infected and the mortality was 3.1 per cent.

Discussion

Theoretically, the value of a pathogen-free isolation unit, such as we have described, in the prevention of infection in patients with hypo-aplasia or aplasia of the bone marrow, could only be assessed after a random trial. In such a trial, alternate patients, taken at random, would be treated either in the P.F.I.U. or by conventional hospital treatment. For obvious reasons, such a trial would seem to us to be impossible. The patients treated in the P.F.I.U. were selected — a selection was necessary because of the limited number of beds, in the P.F.I.U. This selection can only work against the results of the treatment in P.F.I.U. We have in fact admitted to the P.F.I.U. those patients who were hypoplastic before giving chemotherapy and in whom there would have been considerable risk of aplasia during the course of chemotherapy and, consequently, of infection and, in the second group, we have chosen patients who had particularly severe bone marrow aplasia following chemotherapy, which is the reason why there was such a large proportion of the patients who had granulocyte counts of less than 500 per mm^3.

We think that it is possible to make some comparison of the percentage of infection and death from infection amongst patients treated in the P.F.I.U. and those treated by conventional hospitalisation if we limit our attention to acute leukaemia, which is the most homogeneous group of our patients. This comparison is shown in Table 8; there is a very significant difference between the incidence of infection in the two groups of patients: $\chi^2 = 75.0$ for 1 dl, S for P $<$ 0.001, and the incidence of death from infection is significantly lower in the P.F.I.U. (P $<$ 0.06, $\chi^2 = 3.76$ for 1 dl).

Table 8. *Frequency of infection in patients suffering from acute leukaemia*

	In conventional hospital ward	P.F.I.U.
All infections	94/117 (80%)	20/61 (33%)
	$\chi^2 = 75.0$	
Lethal infections	20/117 (17%)	4/61 (6.5%)
	$\chi^2 = 3.76$	

The percentage of infections in patients with acute leukaemia, treated with intensive chemotherapy under normal hospital conditions, although very high, 80 per cent, is still lower than that reported by FREI and his colleagues (1965) when such patients were treated at Bethesda. Comparisons cannot be made with other treatment centres, where the bacteriological investigations have not been carried out in such a systematic fashion.

Our figures, which at the present time are the largest series in the world, for such a clinical trial, have shown the importance of Unit constructed like our P.F.I.U. in diminishing the risk of infection that is inherent in intensive chemotherapy or after prolonged radiotherapy.

It is well understand that at present there is difficulty in comparing the different techniques that can be used to diminish the risk of exogenous infection; in particular, the relative merits of a P.F.I.U. as opposed to isolating the individual by use of the "life island" system that has been tried in the United States (Levitan and Perry, 1968). However, the P.F.I.U. has the advantage of not inducing any psychological disturbance in the patients, as we have shown during the past five years' practice with this system, even when they stay is as long as three months, which could be very difficult in a "life island".

Our results have shown that the most formidable infections which remain in a P.F.I.U. are those due to endogenous organisms, progress needs to be made in this aspect of the problem, for prophylactic antibiotics at present appear to be far more dangerous than effective (Cattan, 1966; Schneider, 1967).

Above all, our results raise the question of the extension of pathogen-free isolation units. It is now evident that all forms of effective anti-cancer therapy have to be intensive, and ought to be carried out in specially constructed P.F.I.U.'s and not in the conventional hospital wards. In the conventional ward, the frequency of infection, sometimes lethal, remains high despite the progress in antibiotic therapy and the symptomatic treatments in the transfusions of leucocytes; these infections always interfere with the pursuit of antimitotic therapy and influence the overall therapeutic results (Cattan, 1966; Schwarzenberg et al., 1966; 1966).

It is clear, at the present time, that a bacteriologist is a key member of any team that wishes to undertake the treatment of malignant disease with the maximum efficiency and the minimum of risk to the patient.

Summary

Since 1965 a pathogen-free isolation unit containing 5 beds has been in use at the Institut de Cancérologie et d'Immunogénétique (Hôpital Paul-Brousse, Villejuif).

The results obtained during the first three years have confirmed the efficacy of this type of unit in reducing the risk of infection in patients undergoing intensive cytostatic chemotherapy, or suffering from granulocytopenia after intensive chemotherapy, or prolonged radiotherapy.

It is therefore desirable that such treatment be carried out systematically in such units. It is now necessary urgently to consider the building of much larger pathogen-free isolation units.

References

Cattan, A.: Le traitement de l'agranulocytose. Presse Méd. 74, 1056 (1966).

Frei, E. III., Levin, R. H., Bodey, G. P., Morse, E. E., Freireich, E. J.: The nature and control of infections in patients with acute leukaemia. Cancer Res. 25, 1511 (1965).

Levitan, A. A., Perry, S.: The use of an isolator system in cancer chemotherapy. Amer. J. Med. 44, 234 (1968).

MacKay, I.: Hexyl resorcinol as an aerial disinfectans. J. Hyg. Camb. 52 (1952).

Mathé, G.: Operational research in cancer chemotherapy. Chemotherapy in the strategy of treatment of cancer. In: Recent Results in Cancer Research, 1 Vol. Ed.: Springer Verlag (in press).

MATHÉ, G., FORESTIER, P.: Un outil moderne de la recherche médicale française, l'Institut de Cancérologie et d'Immunogénétique. Intrications de la recherche expérimentale et clinique. Conditionnement hyposeptique des animaux et malades. Techn. Hospitalière 20, 47 (1965).

SCHNEIDER, M.: Les infections bactériennes et fungiques au cours des leucémies aigues. Sem. Hôp. Paris 43, 438 (1967).

— SCHWARZENBERG, L., AMIEL, J. L., CATTAN, A., SCHLUMBERGER, J. R., HAYAT, M., DE VASSAL, F., JASMIN, C., ROSENFELD, C., MATHÉ, G.: Three years experience of the clinical use of a pathogen-free isolation unit. Brit. med. J. 1969 I, 836.

SCHWARZENBERG, L., CATTAN, A., SCHNEIDER, M., SCHLUMBERGER, J. R., AMIEL, J. L., MATHÉ, G.: La réanimation hématologique. II. Correction des désordres graves des leucocytes et des immunoglobulines. La greffe de moelle osseuse. Presse Méd. 74, 1061 (1966).

— MATHÉ, G., AMIEL, J. L., CATTAN, A., SCHNEIDER, M., SCHLUMBERGER, J. R.: Le traitement symptomatique de l'agranulocytose par les transfusions de globules blancs. Presse Méd. 74, 1057 (1966).

Protected Environments and the Use of Antibiotics

H. E. M. KAY, J. BYRNE, B. JAMESON, and J. LYNCH

The Royal Marsden Hospital, London S.W. 3, England

Several systems of isolation of the infection-prone patient are at present under trial in Great Britain. The units concerned are for transplantation, burns or marrow-depleted patients. In two centres where the isolation depends upon air-flow alone it is too soon to make any assessment except that there appear to be no overwhelming practical difficulties (LIDWELL and TOWERS, 1969; DREWETT and PAYNE, 1969).

Elsewhere cubicle isolation or plastic tent isolators have been used and at the Royal Marsden Hospital it has been possible to make a realistic comparison between these two systems (JAMES et al., 1967; ROBERTSON et al., 1968). The ward at the Royal Marsden Hospital contains seven isolation cubicles with air-filtration and with sterile access via four separate ante-rooms. In addition a single large room has space for two patients in plastic tents which can be connected up to the supply of filtered air.

Both cubicles and plastic isolators depend on the service of a central sterile supply and on a properly equipped kitchen within the ward complex. From the experience of nursing patients in cubicles for a total of about 5000 days and in isolators for 500 days some conclusions can be drawn.

The rate of acquisition of foreign organisms can be substanially reduced by isolation in cubicles. In our ward "apparent" acquisition of staphylococci occurred at a rate of 1.5 per 100 patient-weeks compared with rates of 5 for other wards in the hospital and about 10 in most general hospitals. It should be noted that most of the isolated patients were leucopaenic for part of the time and might be expected to acquire staphylococci more readily. Secondly these were "apparent" acquisitions without a demonstrable source of the organism except in one case. Thirdly the paradox should be emphasised that the apparent effectiveness of isolation is inversely related to the efficiency and resources of the bacteriology department. Comparison by the same laboratory, therefore, is important in a valid assessment of isolation techniques.

Most small children can be nursed satisfactorily in cubicles but, because they have to be picked up, handled and sometimes cuddled, acquisitions of organisms cannot be totally prevented. 100% isolation of older children and adults can, however, be achieved in plastic tents, and we have not hitherto been able to demonstrate acquisition of staphylococci, other bacteria or viruses, in any patient within an isolator. We can conclude that the problems of isolation are essentially solved and that practice is dependent on training and discipline of staff and on economic considerations.

The outstanding problem remains the prevention and treatment of infections by endogenous organisms, particularly those that inhabit the bowel. The most notorious of these is the pseudomonas group but no organism can be considered by itself alone since competition and symbiosis are the bases of a complex ecological system. If one antibiotic-sensitive organism is suppressed or eliminated others, perhaps resistant to antibiotics, may flourish in dangerous abundance. Certain measures appear to be entirely beneficial e. g. the use of hexachlorophane soap to eliminate Staph. aureus from the skin and hair. The case for intestinal antibiotics, however, remains unproven.

We have tried in the past two years to randomise our patients into two groups one of which receives no prophylactic antibiotics; the other group receives Neomycin up to 4 gms. daily, Colistin up to 6 million units daily and Amphotericin B up to 400 mgms. daily. This sounds simple but in practice only about half the treated patients are able to tolerate the doses needed to suppress the bowel flora without getting diarrhoea, nausea, vomiting or other symptoms. In other cases where gastro-intestinal ulceration due to methotrexate or other drugs has occurred we have hesitated to give full doses of neomycin for fear of toxic effects through absorption. At the best these antibiotics may sometimes eliminate one type of Gram-negative organism—we have good evidence of a victory over Pseudomonas in one case but for the most part the organisms can be cultured as soon as the antibiotics are discontinued and have presumably been merely suppressed.

It is possible, however, that even suppression might reduce the risk of acquiring a septicaemia from intestinal bacilli and we have, therefore, compared the incidence of septicaemia in the two groups. The number of cases is small and the groups are, by chance, not exactly comparable as to age and severity of disease but with two septicaemic episodes in 8 antibiotic-treated patients and three episodes in 15 control patients it is clear that the balance of advantage is fairly even. This is a problem that demands a wider trial in a number of different centres.

Summary

Experience over three years in an isolation ward at the Royal Marsden Hospital, where up to seven patients can be nursed in cubicles and two in plastic isolators, has shown that both infection by, and acquisition of, foreign bacteria can be virtually eliminated. Cubicles are the most satisfactory form of isolation for children but plastic isolators, especially in groups, may be more effective and economical for adults.

Infection by endogenous bacteria remains a problem. Preliminary results of a trial with intestinal antibiotics has hitherto shown no significant benefit from this treatment.

References

LIDWELL, O. M., TOWERS, A. G.: Protection from microbial contamination in a room ventilated by a unidirectional air flow. J. Hyg. Camb. 67, 95 (1969).

DREWETT, S. E., PAYNE, D. J. H.: Personal communication, 1969.

JAMES, K. W., JAMESON, BERYL, KAY, H. E. M., LYNCH, J., NGAN, H.: Some practical aspects of intensive cytotoxic therapy. Lancet 1967 I, 1045—1049.

ROBERTSON, A. C., LYNCH, J., KAY, H. E. M., JAMESON, BERYL, GUYER, R. J., EVANS, I. L.: Design and use of plastic tents for isolation of patients prone to infection. Lancet 1968 II, 1376—1377.

Protected Environment, Prophylactic Antibiotics and Cancer Chemotherapy

G. P. Bodey, V. Rodriguez, E. J. Freireich, and E. Frei, III.

The University of Texas M. D. Anderson Hospital and Tumor Institute
Houston, Texas, U.S.A.

With 3 Figures

Introduction and Objectives

Infections are the major cause of morbidity and mortality in adults with acute myelogenous leukemia (AML) [1, 2]. The risk of fatal infection during remission induction therapy approaches 50%. Infection and the threat of infection frequently compromises the administration of chemotherapy. Thus, any program which would substantially diminish the risk of infection should allow for more effective and prolonged administration of chemotherapeutic agents.

The risk of infection is related directly to the number of pathogenic organisms to which the patient is exposed and inversely to host defenses. Germ-free animals are at no risk of infection and, thus, tolerate much larger myelosuppressive doses of total body radiation or chemotherapy [3, 4]. The dose response curve for chemotherapeutic agents is steep. Thus, for the majority of agents, a two-fold difference in dose causes as much as a 10-fold difference in the destruction of neoplastic cells [5, 6]. Thus, effective supportive care in terms of diminishing the risk of infection and hemorrhage should result in an increased proportion of patients who receive an adequate trial (a minimum of six weeks treatment) and from preliminary clinical data, this should increase the frequency of complete remission and increase the duration of unmaintained remission.

The objectives of the protected environment — prophylactic antibiotic program are delineated in Table 1. Most of the efforts over the past several years have related

Table 1. *Protected environment-prophylactic antibiotic program objectives*

Stage 1 Maximally reduce exogenous and endogenous microbial burden
Thereby
Stage 2 Decrease risk of infection in patients with AML
Thereby
Stage 3 Increase patient tolerance of antitumor agents
Thereby
Stage 4 Increase complete remission rate

to Stage I. Continuing studies of prophylactic antibiotic regimens and protected environment units have resulted in increasingly effective programs with respect to reducing the patient's microbial burden. We have attempted to optimize these techniques before proceeding to a definitive therapeutic trial. Thus, most of the following data will relate to the Stage I objectives and qualitative data will be presented with respect to Stage II, III, and IV, objectives.

Results and Discussion

The antibiotic programs that have evolved over the past three years are presented in Table 2. The choice of agent, the dose, cyclic therapy, and other variables have been explored in an effort to define that program which maximally reduces the patient's microbial burden and is well tolerated. Paromomycin, polymyxin B, and gentamicin are primarily effective against aerobic gram-negative organisms, vancomycin is primarily effective against aerobic gram-positive cocci, and anaerobic bacteria, and amphotericin B or nystatin against fungi. Prior to antibiotic administration, the stool contains approximately 10^8—10^{12} organisms per gram and the spectrum of organisms is presented in Table 3. Following the administration of the

Table 2

Oral antibiotics [a]	Dosage	
Antibacterial agents:		
Regimen A		
Paromomycin sulfate	500 mg	
Polymyxin B sulfate	70 mg	
Vancomycin hydrochloride	250 mg	
Regimen B		
Gentamicin sulfate	200 mg	
Vancomycin hydrochloride	250 mg	
Antifungal agents:		
Amphotericin B	500 mg	
Nystatin	3.6 million units	
Topical antibiotics	Concentration in:	
	Spray (cc) [b]	Ointment (g) [c]
Neomycin sulfate	100 mg	5 mg
Nystatin	—	50,000 units
Vancomycin hydrochloride	10 mg	8.33 mg
Polymyxin B sulfate	5 mg	1.66 mg

[a] All antibiotics except nystatin were given in flavored solution every four hours. Nystatin was given at six tablets and 6 cc suspension every four hours. Regimen A or Regimen B was administered with amphotericin B or nystatin.
[b] Applied to nose and mouth four times daily.
[c] Applied to external auditory canals, anterior nares, gums, groin and perianal area four times daily.

18   G. P. Bodey, V. Rodriguez, E. J. Freireich, and E. Frei, III.

Table 3. *Effect of antibiotic regimens on organisms isolated from stool specimens of 6 patients in laminar air flow rooms*

Organism	Total No. isolates	No. of patients with organisms	% of isolates completely suppressed
Aerobic Bacteria			
Bacillus spp.	9	5	100
Citrobacter sp.	2	2	100
diphtheroids	4	4	100
Enterobacter spp.	4	4	100
E. coli	11	5	100
Klebsiella sp.	5	5	100
Lactobacillus spp.	5	5	100
Micrococcus sp.	1	1	100
P. mirabilis	2	2	100
Staph. aureus	1	1	100
Streptococcus spp.	11	6	100
Total	60	—	100
Anaerobic Bacteria			
Bacteroides spp.	9	6	100
Clostridium spp.	14	6	100
diphtheroids	3	3	100
Lactobacillus sp.	1	1	100
Micrococcus sp.	2	2	100
Total	29	—	100
Fungi			
Candida spp.	4	4	75
Geotrichum sp.	1	1	100
Penicilluim sp.	2	2	100
Saccharomyces spp.	3	3	100
Torulopsis glabrata	3	3	0
Total	13	—	69

antibiotic regimen, the bacteria are usually completely suppressed from the stool. Fungi are more difficult to eliminate and *Candida spp.* and *Torulopsis glabrata* may occasionally persist. When such organisms do persist, they usually increase in quantity as other organisms are suppressed [7]. Thus, the antibiotic program affects a billion fold reduction in the microbial burden in the stool, and in approximately 40% of patients studied recently the stools are rendered sterile for periods up to 3 months. When this is not achieved, the persisting organism is usually a fungus.

The antibiotic program for the mouth, throat, and other areas are delineated at the bottom of Table 2. The effect of this program on the organisms in the throat and nose are presented in Table 4. Again, a substantial suppression of organisms is achieved with fungi being the most difficult to eradicate.

The skin constitutes a major portal of entry of infection [8]. In addition to the protected environment and the application of antibiotics to selected areas of the skin (Table 2), the patients received germicidal soap baths and alcohol rinses daily. The effect of this total program on skin microorganisms is delineated in Table 5. In the

Table 4. *Effect of antibiotic regimens on microorganisms*

		% of strains totally suppressed in patients	
		Life Island	LAF Room
Stool	Aerobic	90% (213)	100% (83)
	Anaerobic	98% (90)	100% (42)
	Fungi	51% (37)	67% (18)
Throat	Bacteria	80% (172)	75% (77)
	Fungi	31% (26)	25% (12)
Nose	Bacteria	83% (93)	89% (35)
	Fungi	88% (8)	100% (1)

Table 5. *Median number of organisms cultured from skin during occupancy of Life Island unit (7 patients)*

Site	Week of stay in protected environment			
	Pre-treatment	2	6	12
Scalp	450	B	0	B
Face	900	50	300	50
Neck	1,900	B	B	0
Arms	950	0	B	0
Chest	5,500	0	B	B
Back	50	0	0	0
Abdomen	350	B	0	0
Legs [a]	28,600	B	50	0
Buttocks	1,700	B	B	0
Groin	50,000	50	50	0
Perianal	50,000	900	600	1,500

[a] Total for both.
B = Isolated from Broth Culture only.

Table 6. *Air sampling during patient occupancy*

Site-patient	Number of samples	% Sterile samples	Number organisms recovered/1000 cu. ft. air
LAF room O.W.	11	45	17
LAF room-S.M.	25	56	19
LAF room-B.W.	34	85	2
LAF room-J.P.	32	69	5
LAF room-S.C.	75	72	4
LAF room-H.R.	73	75	6
LAF room-total	250	71	6
LAF corridor	19	5	500
Hospital corridor	5	0	5480
Hospital rooms	15	0	2930

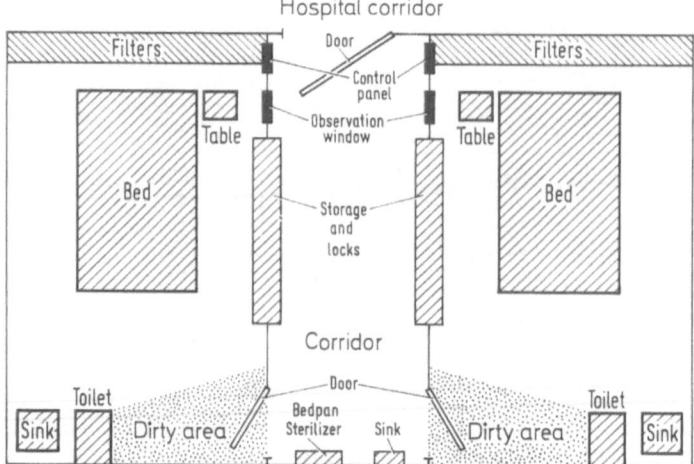

Fig. 1. Floor plan of laminar air flow rooms

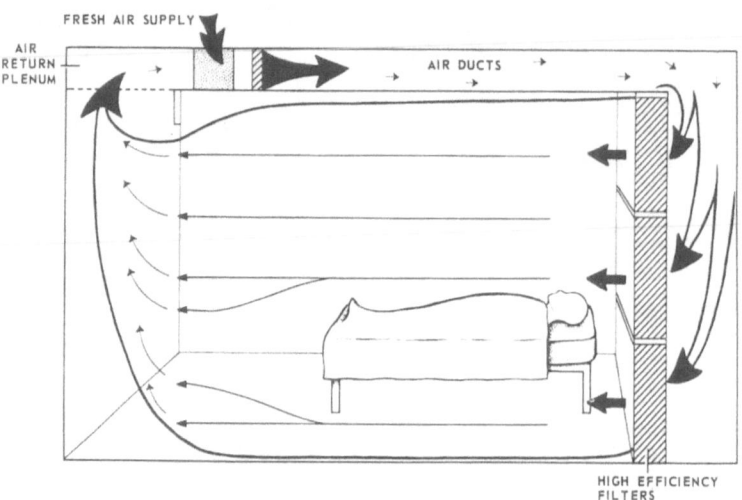

Fig. 2. Diagram of the air supply system in the laminar air flow room. Air passes through the high efficiency particulate air filters and flows in laminar patterns across the room. It returns through ducts in the ceiling

majority of areas of the skin, a marked reduction or elimination of microorganisms is achieved. The perianal area is the major site of persisting organisms on the skin.

During the past 3 years, we have had two Life Islands in operation and over the last 16 months, additionally, two laminar air-flow rooms [9, 10]. Twenty-eight patients have been studied in the Life Island and 10 patients in the Laminar air-flow rooms. The floor pattern, sagittal view and photograph of the laminar air-flow rooms are presented in Figs. 1, 2, and 3, respectively. The details of the development and clinical use of these units have been reported elsewhere [11, 12]. The effectiveness of the laminar air-flow rooms with respect to air contamination is presented in

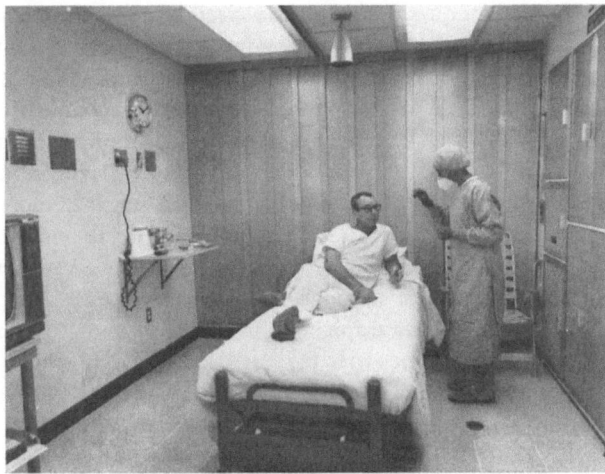

Fig. 3. The sterile attire worn by personnel when entering the clean area of the laminar air flow room

Table 4. Note that in the majority of instances the air samples have been sterile and that the average number of organisms recovered per 1000 cu. ft. air sampled has been only 6. This is in contrast to the normal hospital room which is never sterile and contains on the average of 3000 microorganisms per 1000 cu. ft. of air.

In summary, the use of protected environment and prophylactic antibiotic techniques has rendered a 3 to 10 order of magnitude reduction in both the exogenous and endogenous microbial burden. With the possible exception of fungi, there has been no evidence for a shift in the spectrum to more pathogenic organisms.

The relative effectiveness of the Life Island and the laminar air-flow rooms as compared to control hospital rooms with respect to patient acceptance and microbial burden is presented in Table 7. The control represents 72 patients with AML

Table 7. *Comparison between protected environment patients and controls*

	Control	Life Island	Laminar air flow rooms
Number of patients	72	28	10
Psychological problems	—	6	1
Air cultures			
⁰/o sterile	0	4	71
Organisms/1000 cu. ft	3000	60	6
Floor cultures			
⁰/o sterile	0	70 [c]	67
Organisms/1 sq. ft.	6000	—	50
Adequate chemotherapy [a]	40 (55⁰/o)	26 (91⁰/o)	9 (90⁰/o)
Dose of chemotherapy [b]	1	1—3	1—2
Complete remission rate	25 (35⁰/o)	13 (47⁰/o)	6 (60⁰/o)

[a] Adequate chemotherapy = at least 3 courses (6 weeks).
[b] Dose of chemotherapy = numbers represent multiples of conventional doses.
[c] Cultures of tent surfaces and furnishings.

undergoing remission induction therapy under circumstances where protected environment and prophylactic antibiotics were not administered. Twenty-one percent of patients in the Life Island have had emotional difficulties relating to the confinement whereas only the first of 10 patients entering the laminar air-flow rooms has had such difficulties. The laminar air-flow room approximates much more closely the normal hospital environment whereas the Life Island is more confining. The laminar air-flow rooms are at least as effective and possibly more effective than the Life Island in reducing the patient's microbial burden. In view of this and the fact that the laminar air-flow rooms are more acceptable to the patient, it is our judgment that the development of laminar air-flow rooms should be emphasized.

As delineated in the first paragraph and in Table 1, most of our efforts have been designed to maximally reduce the patient's microbial burden and, hopefully, thereby to increase the effectiveness of chemotherapy. It takes usually six weeks of treatment to produce complete remission in adults with acute myelogenous leukemia. Infections often shorten the duration and compromise the dose of treatment. Thus, the proportion of patients achieving an adequate trial (6 or more weeks of treatment) are an important measure of the risk and presence of infections. Fifty-five percent of control patients had adequate trials whereas 90% of patients in the protected environment-prophylactic antibiotic programs received an adequate trial (Table 8). However, the three groups presented in Table 8 were selected and not randomized.

Table 8. *Protected environment-prophylactic antibiotic program*

	Control	Life Island	Laminar air flow rooms
No. of patients	72	28	10
Psychological problems	—	6 (21%)	1 (10%)
Quantitative air cultures (colonies/1000 cu. ft.)	3,000	45	6 (71%)
Quantitative floor cultures	10,000	—	126 (70%)
Adequate trial (6+ wks. of chemotherapy)	40 (55%)	26 (91%)	9 (90%)
Myelosuppressive chemotherapy (dose)	1	2—5	2—8
Complete remission	25 (35%)	13 (47%)	6 (60%)

Selecting features include primarily the availability of a unit at the appropriate time and patient motivation. Another important selecting feature with respect to the prophylactic antibiotic-protected environment program was the fact that some of these patients had already had remission induction treatment at conventional dose levels and had failed. The complete remission rate for patients in the protected environment-prophylactic antibiotic program was somewhat higher than the control groups (Table 2). Because of the skewed non-random distribution of patients, the significance of the observations with respect to complete remission are questionable. However, they are promising enough to warrant a controlled study. More important are the doses of myelosuppressive chemotherapy tolerated. These relate primarily to arabinosyl cytosine used alone or in combination with cyclophosphamide. The cyclophosphamide dose was twice as high for patients in the protected environment-prophylactic antibiotic setting and further increase was precluded by bladder toxicity. On the other hand, the toxicity of arabinosyl cytosine relates almost exclusively to the bone marrow. In a number of instances, the dose of arabinosyl cytosine to patients in the protected environment was increased by 3 to 8 fold compared to the minimum dose for the control patients. Such treatment resulted in profound and sustained marrow depression. In spite of this, a larger proportion of patients received an adequate trial in the controlled environment (Table 2).

Summary

The immediate objective of this program is to maximally reduce the exogenous and endogenous microbial burden by the application of protected environment techniques and prophylactic antibiotics. The ultimate objective is to reduce the risk of infections in patients with AML and thus increase the effectiveness of antitumor therapy. The immediate objective has been attained in that the microorganisms have been markedly reduced as evidenced by quantitative cultures. Studies designed to further improve the antibiotic program and the protective environment are emphasized. Preliminary analysis would indicate that the risk of infection is substantially reduced as evidenced particularly by the proportion of patients who tolerate at least 3 courses of antileukemic chemotherapy.

References

1. HERSH, E. M., BODEY, G. P., NIES, B. A., FREIREICH, E. J.: Causes of death in acute leukemia. J. Amer. med. Ass. 193, 105—109 (1965).
2. BODEY, G. P.: Infectious complications of acute leukemia. Med. Times 94, 1076—1085 (1966).
3. WHITE, L. P., CLAFFIN, E. J.: Nitrogen mustard — Diminution of toxicity in axenic mice. Science 140, 1400—1401 (1963).
4. WILSON, B. R.: Survival studies of whole-body x-irradiated gum-free (axenic) mice. Radiat. Res. 20, 477—483 (1963).
5. GRISWOLD, D. P., LASTER, W. R., JR., SNOW, M. Y., SCHABEL, F. M., JR., SKIPPER, H. E.: Experimental evaluation of potential anticancer agents. XII. Quantitative drug response of the SA 180, CA 755 and leukemia L 1210 systems to a "standard list" of "active" and "inactive" agents. Cancer Res. 23 (4) Part 2, 271—519 (1963).
6. SKIPPER, H. E., SCHABEL, F. M., JR., WILCOX, W. S.: Experimental evaluation of potential anticancer agents. XIII. On the criteria and kinetics associated with "curability" of experimental leukemia. Cancer Chemother. Rep. 35, 1—111 (1964).
7. BODEY, G. P., LOFTIS, J., BOWEN, E.: Protected environment for cancer patients. Effects of an oral antibiotic regimen on the microbial flora of patients undergoing chemotherapy. Arch. intern. Med. 122, 23—30 (1968).
8. — KIM, Z., BOWEN, E.: A semiquantitative total body skin culture technique for patients in a protected environment. Amer. J. Med. Sci. 257, 100—115 (1969).
9. — HART, J., FREIREICH, E. J., FREI, E., III.: Studies of a patient isolator unit and prophylactic antibiotics in cancer chemotherapy. Cancer 22, 1018—1026 (1968).
10. — Laminar air flow unit for patients undergoing cancer chemotherapy. Germ-free Biology. Plenum Press 1969.
11. — GEWERTZ, B.: Microbiological studies of a laminar air flow unit for patients. Arch. Environmental Health 19, 798—805 (1969).
12. — FREIREICH, E. J., FREI, E., III.: Studies of patients in a laminar air flow unit. Cancer 24, 972—980 (1969).

Studies of Components of Patient Protection Programs: Non-absorbable Antibiotics and Low Bacterial Diets

E. S. Henderson, H. D. Preisler, and I. M. Goldstein

Leukemia Service, Medicine Branch, National Cancer Institute Bethesda, Maryland 20014, U.S.A.

With 1 Figure

Infection is the proximate cause of death in the vast majority of patients with acute leukemia [5, 6, 14] and is the chief cause of inadequate chemotherapeutic trials in drug assessment protocols [2]. Bodey and co-workers have demonstrated a definite correlation between granulocytopenia and infection in patients with acute leukemia [1]. In such circumstances the causative organism is usually found to be a "contaminant" of the skin or gastrointestinal tract. Since not only leukemia per se, but the existing treatments for leukemia regularly induce granulocytopenia, the protection of granulocytopenic patients has for many years been a major concern of leukemia therapists.

Patient protection studies have proceeded in two logical and complementary directions. Granulocyte replacement has been employed in the attempt to correct this major deficiency in the patient's own defense mechanisms. Progress has been slow because of the difficulty in acquiring sufficient granulocytes to repair the vast deficiencies existing in most granulocytopenic patients [4, 13, 15]. The current lack of an effective means to store granulocytes, their short lifespan, and the histo-

Table 1. *Causes of increased incidence of infection in patients with acute leukemia*

I. Complications of the disease
    Granulocytopenia
    Immuno-incompetence including lymphopenia
    Hemorrhage $2°$ thrombocytopenia and/or coagulation defects
    Local leukemic infiltrates, esp mucosal
    Decreased mobility $2°$ malaise
II. Complications of treatment
    Granulocytopenia
    Immuno-incompetence
    Hemorrhage $2°$ thrombocytopenia
    Epithelial injury esp. GI mucosa
    Hypoproteinemia $2°$ GI loss, inanition, defective synthesis
    Exposure to infectious patients and/or personnel
    Exposure to contaminated biologicals, drugs, equipment (e. g. needles).
    Iatrogenic injury e. g. injection sites, marrow aspirations, finger-sticks, etc.

---

compatibility barriers between random donors and recipients combine to reduce the applicability of this approach. As indicated in Table 1 perfection of granulocyte replacement techniques may still not solve the problems of infection in leukemia, since numerous other factors contribute to the initiation and sustenance of microbial invasion in these individuals [7, 8, 14].

The alternate approach has sought to minimize the microbial challenge to the patients's multiply attenuated defense mechanisms by reducing the concentration of microorganisms in his internal and external environment. Most such approaches have combined multiple techniques of asepsis, antisepsis, and antibiosis, in conjunction with some degree of physical isolation [3, 9, 10]. Certain pros and cons of these various procedures are listed in Table 2.

Table 2. *Components of protected environment*

	Advantages	*Disadvantages*
Air filtration	1) Reduction of airbourne microorganisms (exogenous and endogenous) 2) ? Reduction of lower and upper respiratory tract infection 3) Reduction of cross-contamination	1) Expense 2) Discomfort (noise)
Topical antisepsis Skin Upper respiratory tract Mouth Perineal and perianal	1) Reduction of local infection 2) ? Reduction of lower respiratory tract infection	1) Inadequacy of current methods 2) Contact with environment
Gastrointestinal "sterilization" Sterile Diet	1) Reduction of endogenous potential pathogens	1) Expense of preparation 2) Unpalatability
Oral antibiotics	1) Reduction of endogenous potential pathogens	1) Gastrointestinal toxicity 2) Expense 3) Risk of absorption leading to oto-nephrotoxicity 4) Risk of inducing resistant organisms 5) Failure of current regimens to completely suppress fungi
Mechanical isolation	1) Reduction of exposure to exogenous pathogens 2) Reduction of cross contamination	1) Physiological impairment due to confinement 2) Psychological impairment due to confinement 3) Reduction in nursing physician efficacy 4) Expense

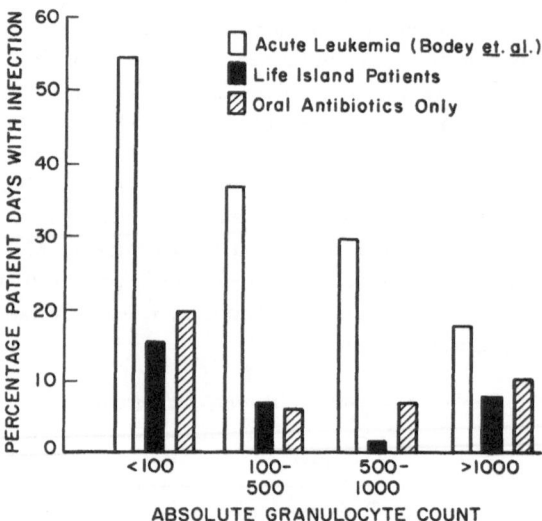

Fig. 1. Comparison of the per cent of days with infection associated with various degrees on granulocytopenia in patients with or without prophylactic protected environment and antibiotics.

Absolute granulocyte counts are expressed as number per cubic millimeter of peripheral blood. Patients in the series of Bodey et al. [1], did not receive prophylactic oral antibiotics, low bacterial diets, or isolation procedures

Since pneumonia is a frequent infection in leukemia [6] there is little reason to suppose that air-filtration by the highly efficient means currently available should not be beneficial. However, it is not practical to apply air-filtration to an entire hospital or even an entire hospital ward, so that some degree of isolation and confinement is required. Laminar air flow room isolation, perhaps the most efficient means of reducing air particle concentrations [11], is unfortunately quite noisy and quite expensive. Less efficient air filtration systems permit contamination through turbulence, and in the case of the widely used "Life Island" equipment, may occasionally increase the concentrates of airborne microbials should the inside of the enclosure become contaminated, or the patient develop a superficial infection.

Topical antisepsis of skin and mucosal surfaces should reduce airborne contamination and the risk of infection developing through local injury, both accidental and incidental to medical procedures. Unfortunately even the most compulsively thorough procedures have been only partially successful in eliminating surface contamination [3, 9, 12].

Suppression of gastrointestinal microflora reduces the body's exposure to microorganisms more than any other measure. This procedure also reduces many of those species, e. g. proteus, E. coli, and pseudomonas, with the highest mortality once systemic infection has occurred. Several regimens combining orally administered, minimally absorbed, broad spectrum antibiotics have been successfully employed [3, 9, 12]. These mixtures have the disadvantage of being in themselves somewhat toxic to the gastrointestinal mucosa. Bacterial suppression has been generally effective, when the drugs could be tolerated, and, in most cases, when autoclaved or

otherwise sterilized food was administered concurrently. Such a program of antibiotics and diet is usually costly and time-consuming to conduct, and may, because
of the decrease in palatability of the diet, aggravate the anorexia or more serious
gastrointestinal discomfort experienced by the patient. These programs are less effective in reducing fungal growth in the bowel [3, 9, 12] and could theoretically induce
microbes resistant to the antibiotics employed.

Some form of mechanical isolation is obviously necessary if organisms are not
to be spread by direct contact with professional personnel or visitors. The disadvantages of isolation are too numerous and obvious to enumerate. Perhaps the two most
important, however, are the restriction of normal activity of the patient resulting
from either the physical or emotional limitations of his environment and the
diminished ascessibility of the patient to his nurses and doctors. All isolator systems
must effect a compromise between these disadvantages and the hoped for reduction
of patient contamination and cross-contamination.

Reports on patient protection programs have not attempted to independently
analyze the contributions, beneficial or detrimental, of the several components of
the system employed. With the possible exception of air filtration the net effect of
any component will reflect the integration of its positive and negative features.
This is particularly the case with mechanical isolation and gastrointestinal sterilization using methods currently available. Certain of these variables are under study
at the National Cancer Institute using the protocol shown in Table 3. Patients with

Table 3. *Current National Cancer Institute patient protection protocol*

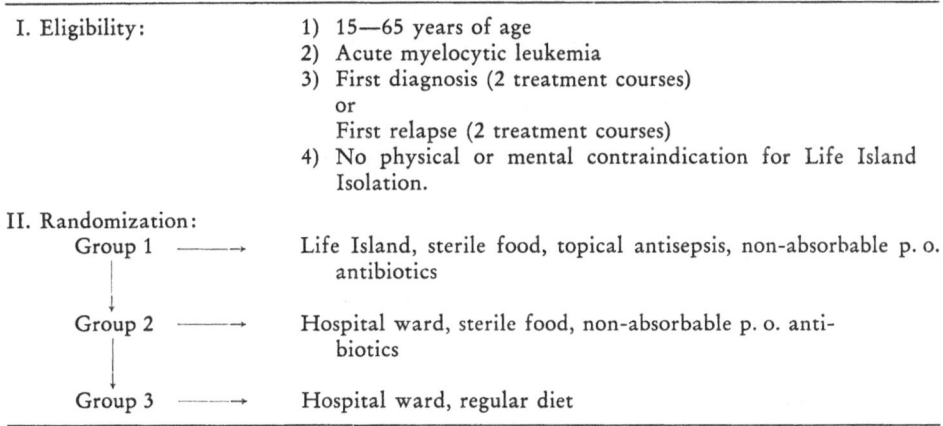

I. Eligibility:	1) 15—65 years of age
	2) Acute myelocytic leukemia
	3) First diagnosis (2 treatment courses)
	or
	First relapse (2 treatment courses)
	4) No physical or mental contraindication for Life Island Isolation.
II. Randomization:	
Group 1 ⟶	Life Island, sterile food, topical antisepsis, non-absorbable p. o. antibiotics
Group 2 ⟶	Hospital ward, sterile food, non-absorbable p. o. anti-biotics
Group 3 ⟶	Hospital ward, regular diet

acute myelocytic leukemia are randomized to 1) the full "Life Island" regimen of
isolation, air-filtration, topical antisepsis, and gastrointestinal flora suppression,
2) gastrointestinal prophylaxis while on a hospital ward, or 3) routine hospital ward
care. It is hoped that this study will indicate which components: air filtration and
isolation or gastrointestinal prophylaxis, will be most likely to benefit an individual
patient, thus identifying the components with maximum current utility, and con-
versely those for which there is the greatest need for further development.

Table 4. *Non-absorbable oral antibiotic regimens employed at the National Cancer Institute for gastrointestinal "sterilization"*

I. Rotating,	7 Drug (rotating)		
Solution A	Bacitracin	15,000 μ/m² QID	Days 1—4
	Phthaly sulfathiazole	0.75 gm/m² QID	Days 1—4
	Neomycin sulfate	0.5 gm/m² QID	Days 1—4
Solution B	Bacitracin	15,000 μ/m² QID	Days 5—8
	Polymyxin B sulfate	12.5 mg/m² QID	Days 5—8
	Neomycin sulfate	0,5 gm/m² QID	Days 5—8
Solution C	Kanamycin sulfate	0,5 gm/m² QID	Days 9—14
	Paromomycin sulfate	0.25 gm/m² QID	Days 9—14
Solution D	Nystatin	250,000 μ/m² QID	
II. Non-rotating,	3 Drug (G-V-N)		
Gentamicin sulfate		200 mg QID	
Vancomycin hydrochloride			
Nystatin		500 mg QID	
		1,000,000 μ QID	

Table 5. *Results of antibiotic regimens used in conjunction with low bacterial diets on gastrointestinal flora of patients with acute leukemia*

Antibiotic regimen	Diet	No. of patients	No. bacteria-free [a]	No. fungus-free [a]
Rotating	Sterile	7	1	2
	Cooked food	4	1	1
G-V-N	Sterile	3	3	0
	Cooked food	6	6	0

[a] No growth in appropriate cultures throughout period of antibiotic administration.

Table 6. *Diets used in National Cancer Institute patient protection studies*

I. Sterile diet
  A. Steam autoclaved meats, vegetables, milk, eggs
  B. Canned Foods
  C. Excludes: salads, fresh fruits and vegetables

II. "Cooked food" diet
  A. Well-done cooked meats
  B. Cooked vegetables and eggs
  C. Coffee, tea, and autoclaved milk
  D. Canned fruits and juices
  E. Excludes: cream, frozen foods, fresh fruits and vegetables, rare meats, raw eggs

III. Regular diet
  A. Standard hospital diet
  B. Fresh fruits, vegetables, pasteurized milk
  C. No exclusions

Concurrent with these studies an attempt has been made to simplify the reduction of the gastrointestinal microflora. The major practical limitations have been the cost and complexity of the drug regimens employed, the unpalatability of both the sterile diet and certain antibiotics, the large expenditure of time and money required in the preparation of sterile diets, and the frequency of administration of the oral antibiotics which interfere with the daily routines of the nurses and the tranquility of the patients especially during the hours of sleep.

First a non-rotating combination of three antibiotics; gentamicin sulfate, vancomycin hydrochloride, and nystatin, given on a QID schedule (Table 4) was substituted for the previously used rotating 7 drug regimen given every four hours. As shown on Table 5 complete bacterial suppression was achieved in every patient for the duration of the simplified antibiotic program. At the dosage employed, i. e. 1,000,000 units QID, nystatin failed to totally suppress fungal growth any patient. Although no patient in this group developed a significant fungus infection, the regimen is clearly deficient in this regard, and larger doses of nystatin with and without supplemental amphotericin B are being investigated. All patients tolerated this regimen well, and while the individual drugs are quite expensive, the reduction in complexity and frequency of administration were economically and psychologically gratifying.

In the hope of simplifying food preparation, the Dietary Department of the National Institutes of Health provided us with meals prepared solely from foods previously found to contain only modest levels of microorganisms. Table 6 contrasts this so called "cooked food" diet with the standard and "sterile" diets employed in our studies. As previously noted (Table 5) results obtained with the "cooked food" diet were indistinguishable from those observed using the sterile diet. The diet, though restricted, is more palatable than the thoroughly sterilized meals at our institution, and its relative ease of preparation permits a several-fold greater productivity of patient protection meals per dietitian.

As shown in Fig. 1 the incidence of infection in granulocytopenic leukemia patients, treated on the open ward with gastrointestinal prophylaxis alone, has thus far been equivalent to the results obtained with patients receiving the full program of isolation, antisepsis, and gastrointestinal prophylaxis. It should, however, be emphasized that these results are not from concurrent, randomized studies and that the "Life-Island" isolators available at present sharply restrict the physical mobility of the patient. Larger air-filtration rooms should minimize the drawback and allow a more accurate assessment of the effects of clean air.

At the same time the demonstration of effective gastrointestinal bacterial stasis and low infection rates obtainable with relatively simple programs of prophylaxis suggests that their wider use may be warranted. There is no way at present to predict the effects of such procedures on the ecology of autochthonous bacteria and fungi, and thus it is obvious that isolation of some sort is to be preferred for all patients receiving antibiotics. These studies further support the important role of intestinal microorganisms on the genesis of infection, and the desirability of further studies to improve means for their suppression. Controlled studies of patient protection programs should, within the near future, provide additional indications of the relative importance of its many components and, as a direct consequence, where the greatest efforts for improvement need be concentrated.

Summary

The high risk of infection in patients with disseminated malignancy receiving chemotherapy has motivated many attempts to minimize exposure of such patients to exogenous and endogenous microflora. Such protective environment regimens include mechanical barriers, air-filtration, and attempts to reduce gastrointestinal bacterial populations by antibiotics and/or low-bacterial diets. The efficacy of gastrointestinal microorganism suppression alone is being evaluated at the National Cancer Institute. Preliminary evaluation indicates a remarkably consistent reduction in gut bacteria following the administration of gentamicin, vancomycin and nystatin by mouth together with either a sterile, or a low bacterial content, diet. Fungal growth was not controlled by this regimen. Clinical trials to date suggest that the incidence of infection in patients so treated is comparable to that achieved when the same prophylactic antibiotic and dietary protocol is combined with mechanical isolation and air-filtration. A randomized controlled study is in progress to more clearly define the relative efficacy of diet, antibiosis, air filtration, and isolation.

References

1. Bodey, G. P., Buckley, M., Sathe, Y. S., Freireich, E. J.: Quantitative relationships between circulating leukocytes and infection in patients with acute leukemia. Ann. intern. Med. **64**, 328—340 (1966).
2. — Hart, J., Freireich, E. J., Frei, E., III.: Studies of a patient isolator unit and prophylactic antibiotics in cancer chemotherapy. Cancer **22**, 1018—1025 (1968).
3. — Loftis, J., Bowen, E.: Protected environment for cancer patients. Arch. intern. Med. **122**, 23—30 (1968).
4. Buckner, D., Graw, R. G., Jr., Eisel, R. J., Henderson, E. S., Perry, S.: Leukapheresis by continuous flow centrifugation (CFC) in patients with chronic myelocytic leukemia (CML). Blood **33**, 353—369 (1969).
5. Han, T., Stutzman, L., Cohen, E.: Effect of platelet transfusion on hemorrhage in patients with acute leukemia. An autopsy study. Cancer **19**, 1937—1942 (1966).
6. Hersh, E. M., Bodey, G. P., Nies, B. A., Freireich. E. J.: Cause of death in acute leukemia. J. Amer. med. Ass. **193**, 105—109 (1965).
7. — Carbone, P. P., Wong, V. G., Freireich, E. J.: Inhibition of the primary immune response in man by anti-metabolites. Cancer Res. **25**, 1177—1181 (1965).
8. — Wong, V. G., Freireich, E. J.: Inhibition of the local inflammatory response in man by antimetabolites. Blood **27**, 38—48 (1966).
9. Levitan, A. A., Perry, S.: The use of an isolator system in cancer chemotherapy. Amer. J. Med. **44**, 234—242 (1968).
10. Mathé, G., Hayat, M., Schwarzenberg, L., Amiel, J. L., Schneider, M., Cattan, A., Schlumberger, J. R., Jasmin, C.: Acute lymphoblastic leukemia treated with a combination of prednisone, vincristine, and rubidomycin. Value of pathogen-free rooms. Lancet **1967 II**, 380—382.
11. Mikelson, G. S., Halbert, M. M., Sorenson, S. D., Vesley, D.: Development of an open isolation system for the care of low resistance hospital patients. August 1968, Final Report Contract PH-43-65-999 NCI, NIH.
12. Preisler, H. D., Goldstein, I., Henderson, E. S.: Gastrointestinal sterilization procedures in patients with acute leukemia. (In preparation.)
13. Schwarzenberg, L., Mathé, G., Amiel, J.-L., Cattan, A., Schneider, M., Schlumberger, J. R.: Study of factors determining the usefulness and complications of leukocyte transfusions. Amer. J. Med. **43**, 206—213 (1967).
14. Viola, M. V.: Acute leukemia and infection. J. Amer. med. Ass. **201**, 923—926 (1967).
15. Yankee, R. A., Freireich, E. J., Carbone, P. P., Frei, E., III.: Replacement therapy using normal and chronic myelogenous leukemia leukocytes. Blood **24**, 844 (1964).

Protected Environmental Rooms in Buffalo[1]

J. F. HOLLAND, B. SAMAL, and J. YATES

Roswell Park Memorial Institute Department of Medicine A
Buffalo, New York 14203, U.S.A.

With 1 Figure

As in other centers where the availability of blood component replacement in acute leukemia has decreased the mortality from thrombocytopenia, infection is the major cause of death in our clinic. Pseudomonas epidemics have occurred on our ward—as on others, and constitute one environmental hazard. Attempts to modify infectious complications by microbial suppression in the patient have moved simultaneously with efforts to provide a pathogen-free environment. The early and pioneering work of MATHÉ and colleagues and BAGSHAWE provide background experience in which medical personnel were surgically garbed to enter the isolation suite. The "Life Island" enclosure of MATTHEWS, Inc., first studied extensively in cancer chemotherapy by the group at the National Cancer Institute in the United States, provided a barrier between personnel and patient, but did so at the expense of eliminating the conventional room structure in which man is accustomed to live.

With support from the National Cancer Institute, we have contracted with the American Sterilizer Company to build two vertical laminar flow protected environmental rooms. Entry is made by medical personnel through pseudopodia which terminate in pseudo space suits of universal size. We have constructed a single room and a room for double occupancy which are located in a special unit together with one "Life Island" enclosure (Fig. 1). The entire ceiling is a laminar flow source and outlet grates in the floor and along the bottom of the walls keep flow laminar almost until reaching floor levels. Room air is recirculated to a ceiling plenum where it is admixed with fresh air and again forced through the HEPA filters at 90 feet/minute. Beds are placed immediately adjacent to a patient care wall in which 2 half suits are placed allowing medical personnel to tend a patient in bed. In addition, there are two full suits attached to the plastic corridors which the attendant pulls behind him into the room as he enters to care for the patient. The suits have their own air supply. The boots are of universal size by using tibial pressure rather than shoe fit. The gloves may be changed without contamination. Medical personnel can enter the pseudopodial suit or the patient care wall suit in 30 to 45 seconds and be ready for patient activities. This is substantially less than the time for donning surgical garb.

[1] This investigation was supported by Public Health Service Research Grant No. Ca-10044 from the National Cancer Institute.

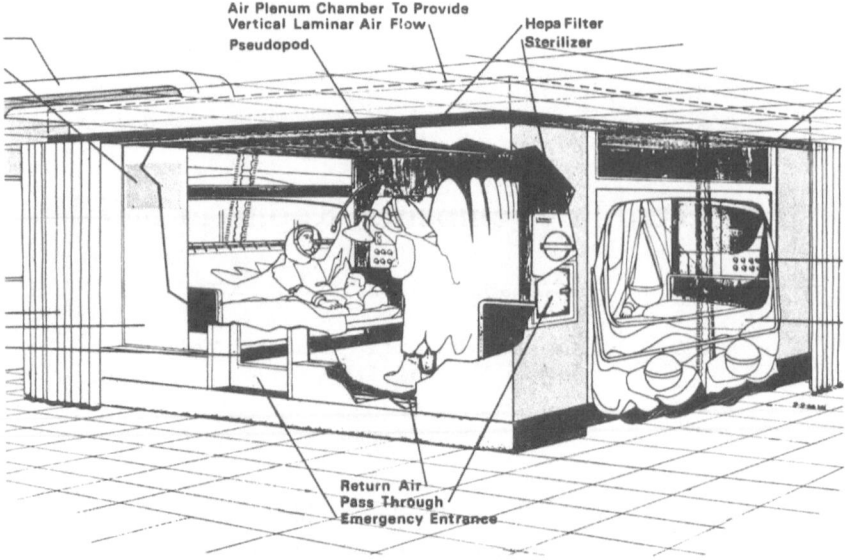

Fig. 1. Plan of double occupancy vertical laminar flow room with personnel in pseudopodia
and at patient care walls

Communication between patient and nurse is accomplished by radio. Parenteral
solutions are kept outside the unit and sterile tubing transverses the wall through
special ports. Autoclaved food and water is passed through ultraviolet locks, and
excreta are passed out.

The patient may be removed from the laminar flow room into an enclosed
sterile cart with its own air filtration system by coupling the cart to a special interface on the wall, sterilization of the interface by peracetic acid and opening of the
cart door and a porthole in the room. The patient may thus be transported to radiation therapy or diagnostic x-ray for such procedures as intravenous pyelography.
Otherwise his entire time is spent in the unit, irrespective of sepsis, until his marrow
function recovers. We keep people in the rooms despite infection assuming that
after its cure there may be less opportunity for another infection to develop.

Psychological reaction to residence in the rooms appears to be somewhat less
stressful than in the "Life Island" enclosure, perhaps in part because the patient has
ready access to walking around in a normally shaped room.

Pre-cleaning of the rooms has been accomplished with washing and topical
antiseptics. Prior to entry, ethylene oxide gas sterilization is practiced. The filtration
system thereafter maintains excellent sterility. Air contamination during occupancy
by patients not receiving antibiotics is minimal, and approximately 2 log orders lower
than the ambient. On most occasions sampled air has been sterile.

Since the rooms are highly efficient for preserving a sterile environment, we have
set about a randomized study of their efficacy in preventing morbidity and mortality
in patients with leukemia. Patients are randomized to care on the open ward, to care
in a single room with full gown techniques for reverse isolation with suppressing
antibacterial drugs and sterile food, or to the laminar flow units with or without gut

sterilization. The antimicrobial drugs are the same for those inside and outside the rooms, and when changed as the state of the art changes, are altered in both. Quantitative surface cultures are made from segmental bath solutions, mouthwash, urine and stool. From the data of the first 11 patients, we believe the possibility exists of proving the value of such a facility. Evaluation of the rooms must be made without the hazard of preselecting patients who are likely to remain uninfected because of relatively well-preserved normal marrow function. If the patient is not infected upon entry, his chances of gaining infection or of mainifesting fever appear to be lower than those infected at the outset. This is sort of a self-proving hypothesis, however, that the sick ones are sicker and the well ones are healthier. We will need a larger experience to determine the value of the various randomization arms for induction of remissions, although it must be recognized that the antileukemic treatments will not remain constant throughout any study. Thus our interpretations will be primarily based on proven infections and fever. The evaluation of the infections of ecological distortion, such as those due to cytomegalic virus, pneumocystis and the fungi will be critical, and may well differ in or out of a sterile environment, with or without attempts to sterilize the body.

We hope our study will remain unbiased and eventually prove in our system whether the concepts of sterile environments and the use of microbial suppression have merit.

Summary

Avoidance of infection is a prime objective for patients with acute leukemia whose bleeding problems are controlled. Environmental containment has been accomplished by constructing rooms with vertical laminar air flow. Personnel approach patients through plastic barriers. This system provides an investigational resource for studying the importance of the endogenous and the environmental flora in causing infection.

The Portable Laminar Flow Isolator: New Unit for Patient Protection in a Germ-free Environment

S. Perry and W. Z. Penland

Clinical Trials, National Cancer Institute, Bethesda, Maryland 20014 U.S.A.

With 7 Figures

It is generally recognized that in spite of antibiotics, infection is one of the major problems confronting the physician in the management of patients with cancer, particularly leukemia. Infection associated with severe granulocytopenia has become the single most important cause of mortality in patients with acute leukemia being responsible for 70% of all deaths (Hersh, Bodey, Nies, and Freireich, 1965; Viola, 1967). Myelosuppression as a consequence of intensive cytotoxic therapy is a major and often limiting factor in the treatment of patients with malignancy. Patients in hospitals receiving therapy with cytotoxic and immunosuppressive drugs are at high risk to infection by a particularly large variety of organisms both endogenous and exogenous. At the present time, one in twenty patients entering a hospital will acquire an infection; this incidence has remained unchanged since the pre-chemotherapy and antibiotic era (Wise, Sweeney, Houpt, and Waddell, 1959; Coriell, Blakemore, and McGarrity, 1968). A recent study at a university hospital demonstrated that approximately one-third of the clinical infections were due to cross infections and two-thirds of these were caused by gram-negative organisms (McNamara, Belows, and Tucker, 1967). From the above considerations, therefore, it seems logical to utilize techniques to protect the patient at high risk to infection from organisms in his environment and at the same time to attempt to reduce his endogenous microbial burden with antibiotics and other means.

Since 1964, the National Cancer Institute has been evaluating a plastic isolator, the Life Island[1], which consists essentially of a modified hospital bed completely enclosed by an air-tight canopy. The unit and the results obtained to date have been well described in the literature and need not be reviewed here (Schwartz and Perry, 1966; Levitan and Perry, 1967; Levitan and Perry, 1968).

Even though the preliminary studies with the plastic film isolator suggest that it is an effective technique for the protection of a patient at high risk to infection, there are a number of problems which limit its usefulness. Occasionally, patients develop minor psychologic disturbances because of isolation in a "fish bowl" environment. Nursing and other paramedical personnel find it physically difficult and

---

[1] Trade mark — T. M. Matthews Research Corporation, Alexandria, Virginia.

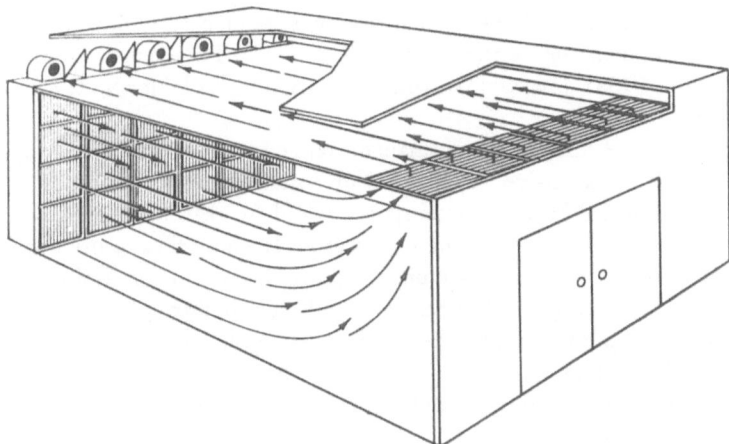

Fig. 1. Diagrammatic representation of a horizontal laminar flow room

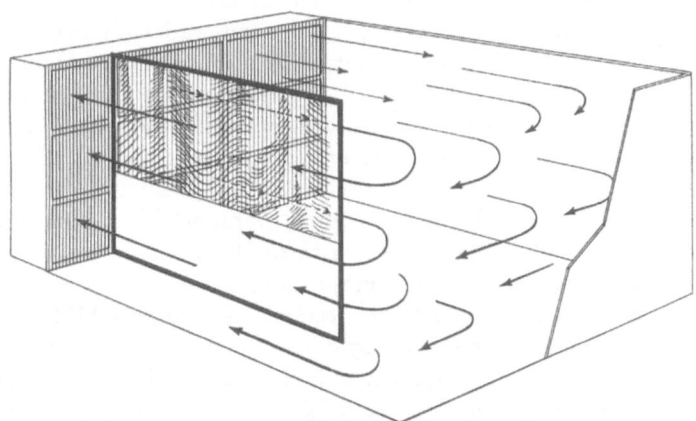

Fig. 2. Air flow in the new portable laminar flow unit

tiring to work with patients in the unit. Cleaning and maintenance are problems, particularly when the unit is occupied by a patient.

For some years industrial firms and government agencies concerned with hardware for space exploration have utilized particle-free rooms for the assembly of space capsules and instruments (AUSTIN and ZIMMERMAN, 1965). The concept utilized in these particle-free rooms, that of laminar air flow combined with high efficiency filtration, has been applied to operating rooms (CORIELL, McGARRITY, and HORNEFF, 1967). MICHAELSON and his coworkers, under contract with the National Cancer Institute, have studied a horizontal laminar air flow room for patients (MICHAELSON, VESLEY, and HALBERT, 1967) and two units based on their studies were recently installed at the M. D. Anderson Hospital. Initial results with patients in these isolators undergoing cancer chemotherapy appear promising in terms of a decreased incidence of infection compared to historical controls. It should be noted, however, that a variety of techniques including air filtration, ultra-violet irradiation, and positive pressure areas have been in use in patient care facilities for some time both in Europe and in the United States (Mathé and Forestier, 1965; Bagshawe, 1964; Lowbury, 1965; James, Jamison, Kay, Lynch, and Ngan, 1967; Voda and Withers, 1966).

Unfortunately, although the permanent laminar air flow rooms appear to be practical, they are expensive to build and install and in addition, restrict the availability of valuable hospital floor space. For these reasons, the National Cancer Institute undertook the development of portable laminar flow units approximately one year ago through a joint effort under contract with Litton Industries, Applied Science Division, Minneapolis, Minnesota. The basic air flow pattern of this isolator differs from contemporary approaches and an example of this difference is shown diagrammatically in Figs. 1 and 2. Key differences include recirculation in a horizontal, not vertical, plane, thereby extending the clean environment and eliminating the need for ceiling ducts.

The first prototype of the portable laminar flow unit is scheduled for delivery early this summer for patient trials at the National Cancer Institute. This unit represents the simplest structural configuration of several possibilities (Fig. 3) and consists of a filter-blower system comprising the end wall with two side walls and ceiling of appropriate plastic panels supported by a modular aluminium framework. The basic structure permits extention of the isolator space in either horizontal direction with the minimum patient floor area measuring $8^1/_2'$ wide $\times 10'$ long (approximately 850 sq. ft.). The overall size of the prototype unit its $11'$ wide $\times 11^1/_2'$ long $\times 7'$ high.

The filter-blower wall is divided into three transportable sections. The smallest section contains polyurethane prefilters and three blower-motor units and is located just outside of the isolator space for purposes of noise control and maintenance. Within the isolator space are two larger sections consisting of HEPA filters which are separated from the blower section by a curtain partition (Fig. 4). This version of the curtain consists of a transparent polyvinyl and polyurethane film with attached flexible plastic gloves that permit patient access and considerable freedom of movement by medical personnel. Thus routine operations can be performed without the necessity of entering the isolator (Fig. 5). In most instances the bed is positioned parallel to the curtain wall with the head of the bed adjacent to the filter bank. Under these circumstances personnel and visitors may enter the unit and as long as they remain "downstream", no contamination will result.

Several features of the prototype unit allow the clinician to evaluate grades and protection as indicated in experimental cancer chemotherapy, burn cases, and with other patients at high risk to infection. Adjustable air flow is possible in the velocity range of 30 to 100 ft./min, thus allowing study of both laminar (minimum turbulence) or diffused air flow effects on airborne contamination. Antibacterial or self-sanitizing plastics, containing such agents as the chlorinated bis-phenols (Davis, 1969), will be incorporated in isolator wall surfaces and in many items of clothing and accessories subject to patient contamination. The contribution of such items to the reduction of pathogenic bacteria and fungi in the isolator environment remains to be studied. Still another feature of these experimental units permits the use of physical barrier walls of plastic film with gloves or alternatively, the use of minimum turbulence air flow as an "air barrier".

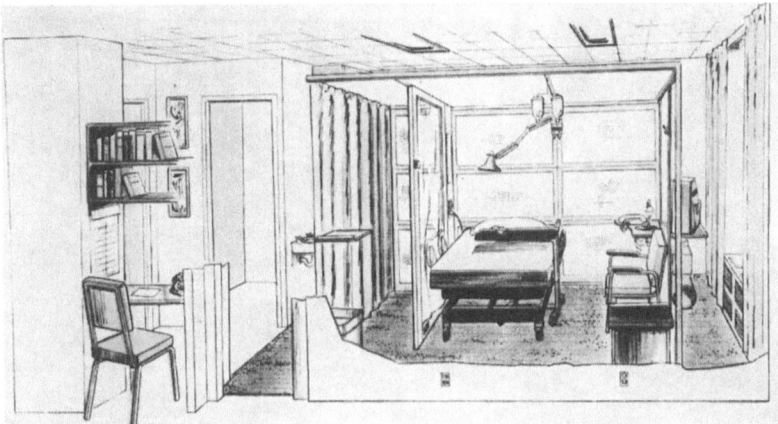

Fig. 3. Portable laminar flow prototype unit. The blower bank is seen on the left and is separated from the patient area by a curtain partition containing openings for gloves. The filter bank is behind the head of the bed

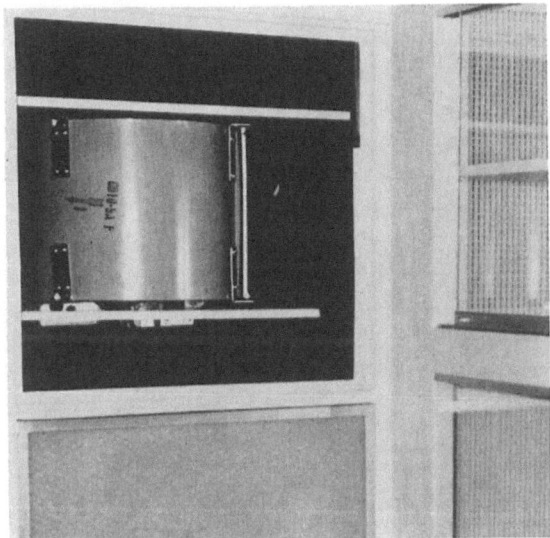

Fig. 4. View of blower housing

The unit can now operate at a noise level approaching 45 decibels at highest in-flow velocities, a level believed to be acceptable in a patient environment. Controls for lighting and air flow are located in the access corridor (Fig. 6). The isolator has an intercom system including a pillow speaker that also allows the patient to control a television, motorized drapes for privacy, room lights, and to communicate with the nurse. The bed is fully adjustable with electrical controls. Water is supplied to a small sink in the interior of the unit utilizing existing hospital room sources. However, the water is sterilized by filtration and ultra-violet and is

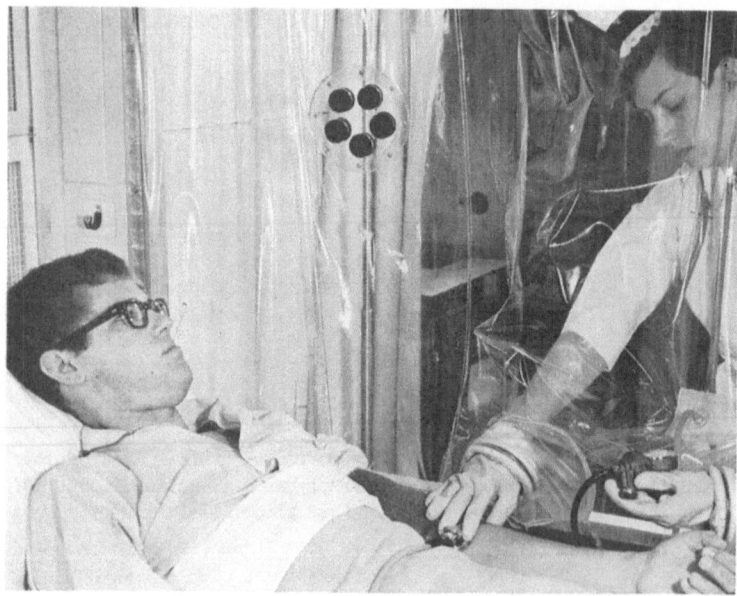

Fig. 5. Nurse working through the plastic gloves attached to the curtain partition

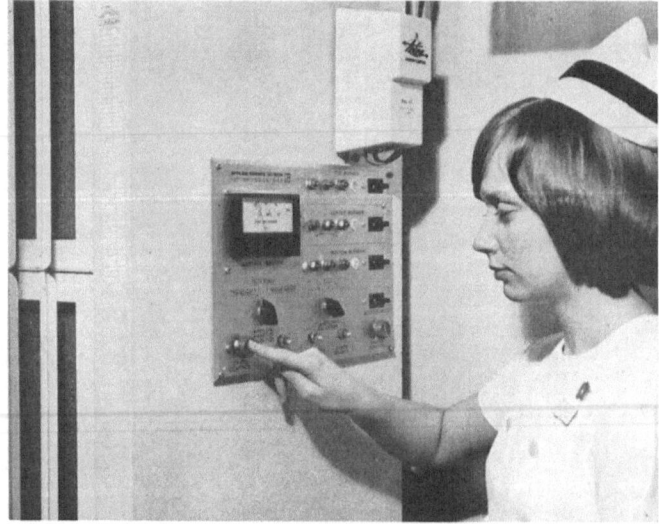

Fig. 6. Controls for lighting and air flow

held in a thermostatically controlled heated reservoir. Several approaches to a compact shower facility are being evaluated, but no final decision has been made. The toilet facility will probably consist of a dual purpose chair with provision for an uncoverable toilet seat and a special disposal container.

Although the initial units are designed for use in single hospital rooms, a great deal of thought has gone into multiple installations for large wards (Fig. 7). The

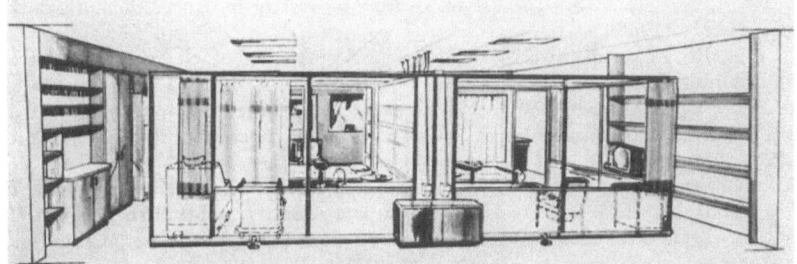

Fig. 7. Two adjacent portable laminar flow units installed in a large hospital room. Two unit installation

design of the portable laminar flow unit is readily altered so that several configurations are possible depending on the location of windows and nursing stations, accessibility desired, etc.

The prototype portable laminar flow units are yet to be evaluated clinically but there is reason to believe that this approach will circumvent most of the objections to both the plastic bed isolators and the permanent forced air isolators. Preliminary hospital surveys indicate that this design will be of great interest to physicians in the management of patients undergoing cytotoxic therapy for malignancy, organ transplants, instances of immunosuppression, and myelosuppression regardless of etiology, and for patients with burns.

Summary

In spite of antibiotics, patients with malignancy undergoing cytotoxic therapy are often at high risk to infection and present difficult problems in medical management. In order to reduce the risk of acquiring infections from the environment, a transportable patient isolator has recently been developed which is now in use in Clinical Trials, National Cancer Institute, Bethesda, Md., U.S.A. It is designed to fit into a standard hospital room and can be installed in 3 or 4 hours. Air enters a filter blower system separated from the patient area by a curtain partition and is then passed through HEPA filters located in the wall behind the head of the bed. The filtered air circulates in a horizontal plane with existing room walls serving as an air return plenum. Sterile water for washing and bathing is provided along with toilet facilities. This isolator has important advantages over existing units aimed at reducing environmental sources of infection.

References

1. HERSH, E. M., BODEY, G. P., NIES, D. A., FREIREICH. E. J.: Causes of death in acute leukemia. J. Amer. med. Ass. 193, 105 (1965).
2. VIOLA, M. V.: Acute leukemia infection. J. Amer. med. Ass. 201, 923 (1967).
3. WISE, R. J., SWEENEY, F. J., JR., HAUPT, G. J., WADDELL, M. A.: Environmental distribution of S. aureus in an operating suite. Ann. Surg. 1948, 30 (1959).
4. McNAMARA, M. J., BELOWS, A., TUCKER, E. B.: A study of the bacteriology patterns of hospital infections. Ann. intern. Med. 66, 480 (1967).
5. SCHWARTZ, S. A., PERRY, S.: Patient protection in cancer chemotherapy. J. Amer. med. Ass. 197, 623 (1966).
6. LEVITAN, A. A., PERRY, S.: Infectious complications of chemotherapy in a protected environment. New Engl. J. Med. 276, 881 (1967).

7. Levitan, A. A., Perry, S.: The use of an isolator system in cancer chemotherapy. Amer. J. Med. **44**, 234 (1968).
8. Austin, P. R., Zimmerman, S. W.: Design and operation of clean rooms. Detroit: Bus. News Publishing Co. 1965.
9. Coriell, L. L., Blakemore, W. S., McGarrity, G. J.: Medical applications of dust-free rooms. II. Elimination of airborne bacteria from an operating theatre. J. Amer. med. Ass. **203**, 1038 (1968).
10. — McGarrity, G. J., Horneff, J.: Medical application of dust-free rooms. I. Elimination to airborne bacteria in a research laboratory. Amer. J. publ. Hlth **57**, 1824 (1967).
11. Michaelson, G. S., Vesley, D., Halbert, M. M.: Laminar flow studies as an aid in care of low resistance patients. Hospitals **41**, 91 (1967).
12. Mathé, G., Forestier, T.: The Institute of Immunology and Oncology, Hospital Techniques **20**, 47 (1965).
13. Bagshawe, K. D.: Ultra-clean ward for cancer chemotherapy. Brit. med. J. **2**, 71 (1964).
14. Lowbury, E. J. L.: Research and control of hospital infections by air-conditioned isolation wards. Nursing **17**, 7 (1965).
15. James, K. W., Jamison, D., Kay, J. E. M., Lynch, J., Ngan, H.: Some practical aspects of intensive cytotoxic therapy. Lancet **1967 I**, 1045.
16. Voda, A. M., Withers, J. E.: Laminar airflow in the OR. Amer. J. Nursing **66**, 2452 (1966).
17. Davis, A. E.: Antibacterial plastics. J. Amer. Ass. for Contamination Control **1**, 63 (1969).

Barrier Nursing of an Infant in a Laminar Cross-flow Bench

J. DE KONING, D. VAN DER WAAY, J. M. VOSSEN, A. VERSPRILLE, and L. J. DOOREN

Department of Pediatrics and the Isolation Ward, University Hospital, Leiden, and the Radiobiological Institute TNO, Rijswijk, The Netherlands

With 4 Figures

Introduction

In patients with severely diminished defence capacities against microbial invasion contamination with pathogenic or potentially pathogenic microorganisms from the environment is frequently followed by infection. Such a defective resistance is present in patients with immune deficiency diseases, in patients treated with cytostatic drugs or ionizing irradiation for hematologic—or other malignancies, in patients treated with immunosuppressive drugs e. g. for organtransplantation, and in patients with extensive skin lesions like large surgical wounds or burns. After contamination of these patients serious infections often can not be avoided in spite of advanced antiseptic and aseptic techniques, immunization and the use of antimicrobial drugs.

As a consequence of the development of gnotobiology and the excellent results obtained in the laboratory with isolation of germfree animals, good isolation techniques became available, and the attention of the medical profession was focused on the possibility of a more or less absolute physical barrier against the contaminated outer world to protect the highly susceptible patient. So "barrier nursing" or "reversed isolation" (the word "reversed" indicating the difference with classical isolation of a contaminated patient) has been developed and steadily progressed especially in the last decade.

In the following we describe the strict isolation of an infant, suffering from Swiss type agammaglobulinaemia, by means of a laminar flow bench. This infant, a five months old boy, was treated successfully by implantation of a fetal thymus and of bone-marrow derived stemcells of a HLA- and ABO-identical sibling. He was nursed under strict isolation conditions until five months after this transplantation. (For details of diagnosis and treatment see [16].)

Isolation Methods

At present there are three kinds of isolation facilities for "barrier nursing".

I. In the "ultra clean" or "pathogen free" isolation ward for reversed isolation [2, 5, 15, 24, 27] the patient is kept in a room under aseptic conditions. Materials are sterilized by ethylene-oxide or autoclaving. Personnel and items enter the ultra-clean room by the way of a double door-lock. The personnel changes to sterile clothes after showering and then dresses with sterile cap, face mask, overgown and overshoes in an entry-lock before entering the patients room. Items pass through locks after double wrapping and sterilization. All items, and ideally the personnel, leave the patients room at the opposite side through a single lock, thus effectuating a one way traffic whenever possible. The air, conditioned for temperature and humidity, is blown into the clean chamber through high efficiency filters and under slight overpressure. Food and drugs are mostly not sterilized. This kind of isolation unit, which may provide a fairly good but certainly not an absolute barrier against exogeneous microbial contamination, is expensive, laborious and personnel-intensive.

II. A more complete physical barrier can be provided by a Trexler type poly-vinylchloride (P.V.C.) isolator, designed and used for rearing of germfree animals [30] and modified for patient isolation. Personnel remains outside the isolator, handling the patient by means of gloves. Air enters under overpressure through a high efficiency inlet filter, and leaves through a fluid trap or an outlet filter. Items are passed through a lock, which is kept as clean as possible by either ultraviolet lamps, and/or an outward high velocity stream of filtered air, or through a germicidal trap. [22]. Results obtained with this method of isolation with a mechanical barrier between patient and outside world are good [3, 4, 17, 18, 19, 28]. However, nursing of an ill patient by means of gloves remains cumbersome and time consuming. Furthermore the psychological problems for the patient during a stay in this kind of isolator, without the possibility of leaving the isolator or even the bed, must not be underestimated.

III. Since a few years so-called "laminar flow" rooms are in use for barrier nursing of patients. In these rooms a continuous horizontal (cross flow) or vertical (down flow) stream of filtered turbulence-free air exists. The "laminar flow system" was developed for the U.S.A.-space project and is in use since in many different branches of industry. According to U.S. Federal Standard 209 a the room was rated "class 100", if the number of particles measuring 0,5 μ or larger did not exceed 100 per cu. feet of air. The air is filtered by so-called high efficiency particulate air (HEPA) filters, which trap 99,97% of particles measuring 0,3 μ and larger as tested with the dioctylphtalate (D.O.P.) test. By multiple microbiological studies it was shown that the air in laminar flow rooms was free of bacteria [1, 10, 11, 12, 32] and even of viruses [25]. These findings led to the application of the laminar flow principle in pharmacy, in microbiological laboratories [20, 29] and in medicine [14, 21, 23, 34]. The application of laminar flow in barrier nursing has two advantages above the blowing of filtered air in standard cubicles. Firstly the concentration of microorganisms in the air at the patient's site is extremely low because of the high turnover and the use of sterile air. The only source of contamination of the air in the area of the room is the patient disseminating his own flora. Secondly dust and microorganisms disseminated by the personnel remaining down stream of the patient will not reach the patient because of the one way direction of the airstream.

A Laminar Flow Bench for Reversed Isolation of an Infant

In december 1968 a five months old boy with Swiss type agammaglobulinaemia was successfully treated by bone-marrow transplantation [16]. In view of the good results of the use of a laminar flow bench for prevention of contamination and cross-contamination in germfree and antibiotic decontaminated animals [31] we decided to isolate this highly susceptible infant in a laminar flow bench. This isolation was started before transplantation treatment and was continued until five months thereafter. The bench used was an industrial laminar flow bench, with inner dimensions of 1.78 m length, 0.57 m height and 0.61 m depth [1]. The unit was equipped with an ultra HEPA filter with an efficiency of 99.997% for particles of 0.3 μ and larger [2], as checked by the manufacturer with the di-octyl-phthalate (D.O.P.) test [13]. The prefilter was made from washable industrial foam plastic. Air flow was maintained by one high capacity, slow speed, direct drive blower. Light was provided by three separately switchable fluorescent lamps above an opal perspex ceiling panel. The two sidepanels were made of clear perspex. The air temperature inside the bench could be raised 2.7° C above the temperature of the inlet (recirculated) air, by two heating elements, with a capacity of 1 KW each, placed in the outflow tract of the blower. The rotation speed of the blower, and by this way the air velocity in the bench, was adjustable by means of a variac. Two manometers indicated the pressure drop over prefilter and ultra HEPA filter.

For the purpose of adequate nursing of an infant several modifications of and additions to this industrial bench were necessary (Figs. 1 and 2). The working table was raised 7 cm and the inside depth was changed from 61 to 80 cm. As a consequence of this enlargement the ceiling was extended by a perspex hood and the perspex side walls were enlarged. One of these was provided with a standard type cylindrical entry lock (29 cm in diameter) made of perspex, which could be closed with a plastic cap on each side. To this entry lock either a transport (Figs. 3 and 4)— or a storage isolator could be connected by interposing a P.V.C. tube, which could be sterilized by spraying of 2% peracetic acid. Thirty minutes after spraying the cap at the side of the bench was removed and the P.V.C. pass-through was dried with a sterile cloth, followed by the removal of the other cap. The front opening of the bench, with the exception of the lowest 10 cm part, could be closed by a transparent perspex front panel [9] which made it possible to reduce the air velocity of 50 cm per sec. inside the bench with approximately one third. This modification did not disturb the laminar airflow pattern inside the bench as tested with the tetanium tetrachloride vaportest. When the bench was operated with reduced flow the noise level was remarkably decreased. The perspex front panel was provided with two neoprene gloves, of the type used in a P.V.C. isolator. To prevent contamination of the gloves during opening of the front panel, the apertures of these gloves could be closed by rotating plastic covers. The infants' bed was especially designed for use in this laminar flow bench with removable front and sidewalls and with dimensions calculated as to prevent the infant climbing over or falling out.

For regulation of the temperature a thermostat was placed at the outlet side of the bench and connected with the heating element. It appeared necessary to set the thermostat at 25° C to maintain a normal body temperature of the infant. The laminar flow bench was placed in an ordinary hospital cubicle recirculating the air inside. Because this cubicle was not provided with air-conditioning, the control of the humidity of the air inside the bench gave some problems. Two water nebulizers

---

[1] Bassaire 6 ft. "laminair" flow clean air bench unit, John Bass Ltd., Fleming way, Crawley, Sussex, G.B.

[2] Mine Safety Appliances Company, Pittsburgh, Pa. 15208, U.S.A.

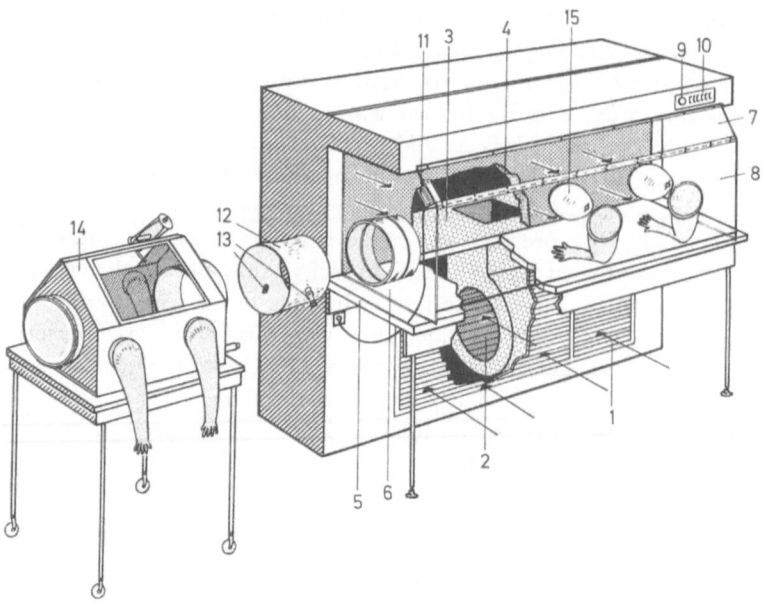

1) Prefilter
2) Blower
3) Supply plenum
4) HEPA-filter
5) Working table
6) Perspex sidewall with entry lock
7) Perspex hood
8) Perspex frontpanel, with neoprene gloves

9) Regulation of blower speed
10) Switches for lights and heating element
11) Thermostat
12) P.V.C. tube
13) Nipples for peracetic acid spraying
14) Storage isolator
15) Plastic cover of glove opening

Fig. 1. Schematic drawing of the laminar cross flow bench and the storage isolator

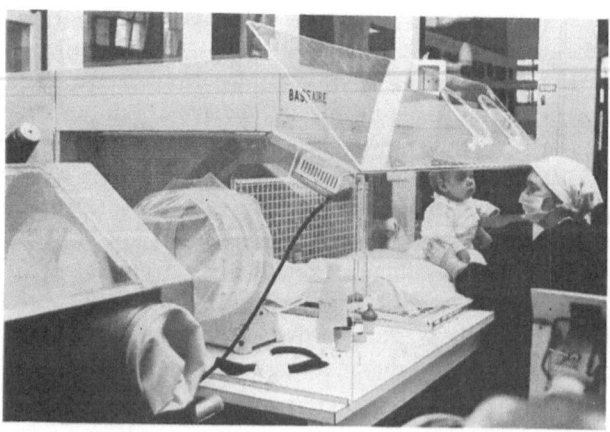

Fig. 2. The patient in the laminar flow bench, visited by his mother

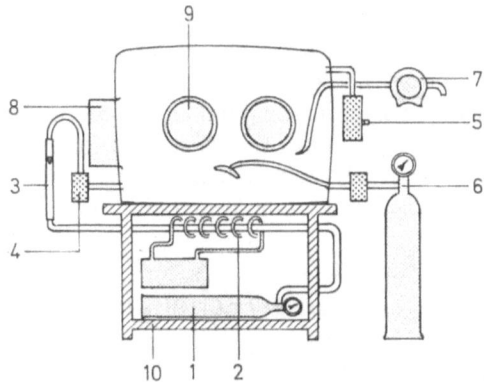

1) Cylinder with compressed air
2) Heating element
3) Flow meter
4) Inlet filter
5) Outlet filter

6) Oxygen line
7) Suction line
8) Pass-through
9) Neoprene gloves
10) Trolley

Fig. 3. Schematic drawing of the P.V.C. transport isolator

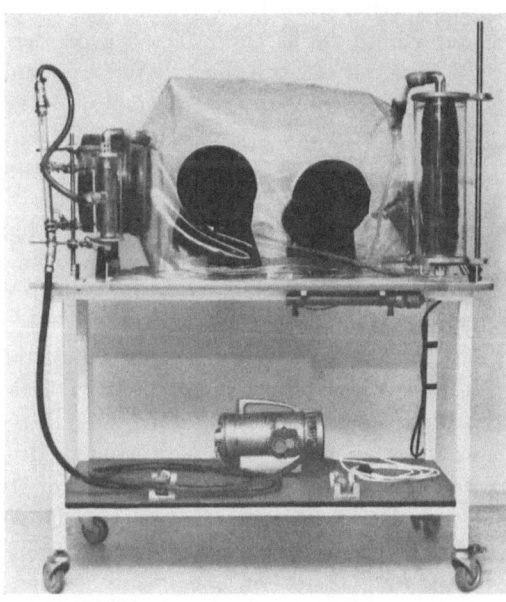

Fig. 4. The P.V.C. transport isolator. For the transport of the patient as described, the isolator has been simplified by removal of the heating element, the oxygen line and the suction line, whereas the compressed air cylinder was exchanged for a compressor

were continuously in use inside this cubicle. Regular bacteriological control and regular sterilization of these nebulizers were performed. In this way the humidity of the airstream at the outlet side of the bench could be maintained at circa 40%, as continuously checked by a hygrometer. Humidification of the air with steam gave difficulties as this caused too high rise of the room temperature.

The air velocity was regularly measured by means of an anemometer, whereas the airflow pattern was checked with titanium-tetrachloride-vapor.

Nursing Technique

After the blower of the bench had been running for at least 12 hours, the inside of the bench was cleaned and sterilized by spraying of 2% peracetic acid solution on the walls and the bed. After another half a day the mattress, wrapped in plastic and sterilized also with peracetic acid, was introduced. Linen, diapers and clothes were sterilized with ethylene oxide and were introduced also through the open front side. The plastic bags, containing the items, were opened in the stream of sterile air in front of the bench by a nurse. The contents were then taken out by another nurse dressed with a face mask, cap, sterile gown and sterile gloves.

The infant, during the first weeks after admission being nursed in an isolation ward, was dressed in sterile clothes and placed in a P.V.C. transport isolator (Figs. 3 and 4), previously developed and used for transport of a newborn infant after germfree delivery. After connection of this transport isolator to the laminar flow bench, the connecting P.V.C. sluice was closed with caps on both ends and sterilized by the spraying of 2% peracetic acid. After 30 min the sluice was opened on the bench side and wiped out with a sterile cloth. The cap on the other end was then opened and the infant was passed through. For all further manipulations inside the bench common surgical aseptic procedures were employed. Persons handling the infant were dressed with caps, masks, sterile overgown and sterile gloves. All other persons entering the cubicle, like nurses assisting with the aseptic procedures, used clean gowns, caps and masks to minimize the amount of bacteria and dust. For daily routine nursing of the infant the frontpanel of the bench was opened by an assisting nurse after increasing the airvelocity to 50 cm per sec. The front part of the working table was cleaned with 70% alcohol. All items to be brought in were sterilized either by ethylene oxide or by autoclaving: linen, clothes, toys, comb, basin, scale, feeding bottles, teats etc. Medical and laboratory instruments e. g. stethoscope, and connecting cables e. g. for electrocardiography, temperature measurements etc. were also sterilized by ethylene oxide. Presterilized disposable materials were used as much as possible. Bottles with sterile water and bottles with condensed milk, heat treated in the factory and garanteed except for sporeformers, were firstly cleaned and then sterilized at the outside by placing them in a plastic bag, into which 2% peracetic acid was sprayed after closing the bag thoroughly. The formulas for the infant were prepared inside the bench using these two ingredients. Drugs were not sterilized except for the outside of the bottles. A stock of bottles with water and with condensed milk and eventually of other items such as drug bottles, was kept in the connected autoclavable stainless steel storage isolator. When the infant grew older and needed cereals and vegetables these were "sterilized" in a pressure cooker.

For radiological examination of the infant the storage isolator was disconnected and replaced by the P.V.C. transport isolator. The sterilization of the connecting lock was done as described above, and the infant was then transported in this plastic isolator to the X-ray department. X-rays were taken through the P.V.C. wall with good results.

Microbiological Control of the Isolation Barrier

Slitsampling at two-weekly intervals inside the cubicle in which the bench was placed indicated that the air contained 9—15 microorganisms per m³, which number rose to 17—52 per m³ during handling and bathing of the infant, when 3 persons were inside the cubicle. The air of the ward outside the cubicle contained 250—400 microorganisms per m³. Recirculation of the air through the bench evidently reduced the number of microorganisms in the air of the surrounding cubicle by a factor 10 to 25.

During the nursing of the infant the efficiency of the isolation barrier was checked by direct follow up of the patients' microbiological flora. Three times a week swabs were taken from the infants' nose, throat, ear, axilla, groin and faeces for bacteriological culture. Once weekly a throatswab and faeces were taken for isolation of respiratory- and enterogenic viruses. Regularly also bacteriological cultures were performed from feedings and drugs. At the time the boy entered the laminar flow bench his flora consisted of: Escherichia coli, Staphylococcus albus, enterococci, Streptococcus viridans and Candida albicans. During his stay of five months in the bench other potentially pathogenic bacteria were found either once or very transitory. Pathogenic bacteria like Staphylococcus aureus, Streptococcus haemolyticus, Haemophilus influenzae, pneumococci, Pseudomonas were never cultured from the infant. Respiratory- or enterogenic viruses were also not isolated during his stay in the bench.

After discharge of the patient and after sterilization of the bench, eight cages, each with two germfree mice, were introduced through the entry lock and placed at various sides in the bench. The animals were kept there for 17 days with the frontpanel of the bench closed, and for another 15 days with the frontpanel opened. All bacteriological cultures of the faeces were sterile, and after 32 days the mice were still completely negative.

Influence of Air Flow and Air Exchange on the Thermal Regulation and Fluid Balance of the Infant

In order to obtain information about the amount of water loss and about the thermoregulatory mechanisms of the infant under the climatic conditions of the laminar flow with its high air-exchange, the humidity and the temperature of the air inside the bench were measured, as well as the boys' skin temperature at different sites and the temperature of the inner side of the cabinet wall. During these investigations the patient was wearing a double layer of cotton clothes, which covered his breast, abdomen, back and arms, while his face, hands, legs and feet were unclothed. He was sitting with flexed knees, playing quietly with some toys. Because of the strict isolation barrier more elaborate measurements like metabolic rate of the infant and water loss by evaporation were not possible. With the use of the results of these measurements and of some literature data we calculated heat loss by radiation to be approximately between 5.7 and 7.0 KCal per hour and heat loss by convection to be 9.0—12.0 KCal per hour (see addendum). Accepting for this infant a calculated metabolic rate of 22.0 KCal per hour, heat loss by evaporation could be estimated as between 3.0 and 7.3 KCal per hour or 14—33% of the total heat loss. Water loss by evaporation was calculated as 5—13 ml per hour (see addendum). These findings can be considered as quite normal and lead to the conclusion that the climatic conditions in the laminar flow bench most likely did neither influence the metabolic rate of the infant by excess cooling, nor the water-balance by excess sweating. This was confirmed by the excellent clinical condition of the infant. Never was an excess of sweating, or of shivering observed, while the core temperature, the water intake and the urinary output were quite normal.

Discussion

Our results show that an infant can be protected effectively against contamination with either potentially pathogenic or pathogenic bacteria or viruses from his environment by nursing him in a laminar flow cabinet. No adverse effects on the infant were noticed. The easy accessibility of the boy was appreciated by the personnel and not the least by his parents, because it gave the opportunity for a good affective contact. During the months of isolation the boy showed a quite normal psycho-motor development, stimulated among else by daily visits of the physical therapist. For the handling of the infant two nurses were needed, one in sterile dress and one for assistance. They were very quickly accustomed to this nursing technique. It appeared that for the proper performance of this task, including e. g. preparation of materials for sterilization etc. the routine nursing staff of this paediatric ward had to be increased with one extra nurse during 15 hours per day assisted by a second extra nurse during 4 hours per day. Because the laminar flow unit took the place of one ordinary bed in the ward, and because the infant was in good condition needing only routine paediatric nursing care, this extra-staff can be considered as being needed for the operation of one laminar flow unit. In case the patient needs intensive care more staff will be needed.

It will be clear that in order to achieve a good isolation by means of a laminar flow bench, apart from very careful personnel, several facilities are essential, like sterilization by either ethylene-oxide or autoclaving, room for storage of the numerous sterilized items, and good bacteriological and virological laboratory facilities. A separate isolator, connected with the bench, is necessary for storage especially of bottles sterilized at the outside by peracetic acid, and to keep the infant temporarily e. g. during transport. A separate storage- and a transportisolator were used in this case, but these two can surely be combined.

Several technical improvements of the described unit can be suggested. Air velocity should be regulated automatically e. g. during opening of the frontpanel and in case of increasing resistance of the filter by plugging. Two blowers, on different power blocks, should function together, each of them automatically generating the full airflow if the other one fails. Temperature and humidity of the air inside the bench should be regulated automatically after being adjusted. An alarmsystem for temperature, humidity, air velocity and electrical power is necessary. A good solution for the weighing of the patient has still to be found, as well as for the supply of sterile oxygen and for the passing of the isolation barrier by the connections of infusion systems, monitoring apparatus, artificial respirators, suction apparatus etc. In older children the sterilization of the diet still offers a problem.

If by means of this laminar flow system an absolute protection against contamination with microorganisms from the surroundings can be achieved, the way is opened to selective or complete decontamination of a highly susceptible patient to safeguard him against endogenous infections [31, 32].

Addendum

Data list

Data of the Patient

Age: 9 months.
Length: 74 cm.
Weight: 8350 grams.
Total surface area: 0.4 m², according to Dubois' formula.
Effective area in   0.3 m², about 75%/o of total surface area (WINSLOW et al.,
   sitting position: 1949).
Metabolic Rate: 22.0 KCal hour^{-1}. This value was calculated for sitting position as 1.16 times (BROCK, 1954 a) a Basal Metabolic Rate of 19 KCal hour^{-1}, which is the mean value of 4 different literature data (BROCK, 1954 b).

Temperature in °C.

Area	Ratio $\frac{\text{special area}}{\text{total area}}$	Temperature of the skin	Temperature of the surface
Feet	0.07	31.7	31.7
Legs	0.26 [a]	31.7	31.7
Breast and Abdomen	0.18	32.8	31.4
Back	0.17	34.5	32.5
Arms	0.14	32.7	31.4
Hands	0.05	32.5	32.5
Head	0.13 [a]	34	34
Average value		32.9 [b]	32.1 [b]

[a] For adults these fractions are respectively 0.33 and 0.07. In children these ratios are different, because the length ratios differ (BROCK, 1954 c).
[b] These average values were calculated according to: 0.07×feet temp.+0.26×leg temp. +etc.+0.13×head temp.

Data of the Bench

Mean temperature of
   the cabinet wall: 28.7° C.
Air temperature: 28.2° C.
Air humidity: 36%/o is 10.3 mmHg.
Air velocity: 30 cm sec^{-1}, according to the qualifications of the manufacturer.

Calculated Heat Loss by Radiation (H_r)

$H_r = Ar \, Kr \, (Tw^4 — Ts^4)$ is the general equation of Stefan Boltzmann to calculate heat loss by radiation.

H_r is the heat transfer in KCal hour^{-1}, which is positive if heat is gained and negative if heat is lost (Ts > Tw).

A_r is effective surface area of radiation (0.3 m^2, see Datalist).

K_r is an universal constant factor of $4.92 \cdot 10^{-8}$ KCal hour^{-1} (Winslow et al., 1949).

Tw is the average value of wall temperature in degrees Kelvin: $273 + 28.7$ (see Datalist) $= 301.7°$ K.

Ts is the average surface temperature in degrees Kelvin: $273 + 32.1$ (see Datalist) $= 305.1°$ K.

These data give a heat loss by radiation $H_r = 5.7$ KCal hour^{-1}. However if we use for the calculation an average surface temperature equal to the average skin temperature Ts $= 273 + 32.9$ (see Datalist) $= 305.9°$ K, then the data give a heat loss by radiation $H_r = 7.0$ KCal hour^{-1}. Only if the double cotton layer is a complete isolator for radiation we have to take into account the value 5.7 KCal hour^{-1}. Most likely the real value for heat loss by radiation is between 5.7 and 7.0 KCal hour^{-1}.

Calculated Heat Loss by Convection (H_c)

$Hc = Kc \, Ac \, \Delta T$ is the equation we have used for calculation of the heat loss by convection (Ruch and Patton, 1965).

K_c is the convection coefficient which is about 8.5 KCal m^{-2} hour^{-1} °C^{-1} (Ruch and Patton, 1965).

A_c is the effective heat exchange area of 0.3 m^2 (see Datalist).

ΔT is the temperature difference between body surface and air.

If we accept an average surface temperature of 32.1° C as the real temperature for the calculation of the heat loss by convection then $Hc = 9.9$ KCal hour^{-1}. However if we take into account the average skin temperature of 32.9° C the heat loss $Hc = 12.0$ KCal hour^{-1}. The double cotton layer is not an airtight clothing. This means that air is blowing a little between clothes and skin. So the calculated value $Hc = 9.9$ KCal hour^{-1} is very probably too low. But it may be sure that the air velocity near the covered skin is not 30 cm sec^{-1}, so for this skin area Kc of 8.5 is too high. Total heat loss by convection will surely be less than 12.0 KCal hour^{-1}. If on the other hand we use the formula $Hc = Ac \, \Delta T \sqrt{V}$, in which V is the air velocity in feet per minute (60 ft. min^{-1}), then the calculated heat loss by convection is between 9—11 KCal hour^{-1}. Combining these two calculations, the range of heat loss by convection may be 9.0—12.0 KCal hour^{-1}.

Heat Loss by Evaporation H_e

Heat loss by radiation may be 5.7 < Hr < 7.0 (KCal hour^{-1}) and heat loss by convection 9.0 < Hc < 12.0 (KCal hour^{-1}). Heat loss by evaporation (He) can then easily be calculated by subtracting the sum of these values from the metabolic rate of 22 KCal hour^{-1} 3.0 < He < 7.3 (KCal hour^{-1}). Because the wall of the bench is a good isolator and moreover the patient was sitting on a thick foam mattress, we assumed a heat loss by conduction near to zero. So heat loss by evaporation seems to be in the range of 14—33% of the total heat loss, which is a quite normal situation. Even if we accept a metabolic rate of 1.3 times BMR, the heat loss by evaporation is quite normal (23—40%).

Water Loss by Evaporation

This can easily be calculated from $\dfrac{He}{0.58}$ ml hour^{-1}, which is in this case between 5—13 ml hour^{-1}.

Summary

A five months old infant, suffering from Swiss type agammaglobulinaemia, was strictly isolated during 5 months by means of nursing in an modified industrial type laminar cross flow bench. During this period no contamination with pathogenic bacteria or viruses from the surroundings was noted. This isolation procedure therefore appeared to be effective, whereas it was also rather easily operated in a routine paediatric ward. A full description of the apparatus and the nursing technique are given and suggestions for further improvements are described.

Acknowledgment

We thank Dr. J. B. Wilterdink, Department of Microbiology, University Hospital Leiden, for virological studies, and Dr. M. J. van Toorn, Department of Microbial diseases, University Hospital Leiden, for supervision of bacteriological studies. We also thank the nursing staff, Department of Paediatrics, University Hospital Leiden, for their great help and devotion.

References

1. Arnold, V. E., Jack, A. J., King, J. G., Marsh, R. C., Whitfield, W. J.: Preliminary report on microbiological studies in a laminar down-flow clean room. Research report Sandia Lab., Albuquerque, Febr. 1965.
2. Bagshawe, K. D.: Ultra-clean ward for cancer chemotherapy. Brit. med. J. 9, 871 (1964).
3. Barnes, R. D., Tuffrey, M., Cook, R.: A "germfree" human isolator. Lancet 1968 I, 622.
4. Bodey, J. P., Hart, J., Freireich, E. J., Frei, E.: Studies of a patient isolator unit and prophylactic antibiotics in cancer chemotherapy. Cancer 22, 1018 (1968).
5. Bowie, J. H., Tonkin, R. W., Robson, J. S., Dixon, A. A.: The control of hospital infection by design. Lancet 1964 II, 1383.
6. Brock, J.: Biologische Daten für den Kinderarzt, Bd. II. Berlin: Springer 1954 a. S. 438.
7. — Biologische Daten für den Kinderarzt, Bd. II. Berlin: Springer 1954 b. S. 401.
8. — Biologische Daten für den Kinderarzt, Bd. I. Berlin: Springer 1954 c. S. 93.
9. Cook, R.: Personal communication, 1969.
10. Coriell, L. L., McGarrity, G. J., Horneff, J.: Medical applications of dust-free rooms. I: Elimination of airborne bacteria in a research laboratory. Amer. J. publ. Hlth 57, 1824 (1967).
11. Decker, H. M., Buchanan, L. M., Hall, L. B., Goddard, K. R.: Air filtration of microbial particles. Amer. J. publ. Hlth 53, 1982 (1963).
12. Favero, M. S., Puleo, J. R., Marshall, J. H., Oxborrow, G. S.: Comparative levels and types of microbial contamination detected in industrial clean rooms. Appl. Microbiol. 14, 539 (1966).
13. Firman, J. E.: High efficiency air filtration. Filtr. and Separ. 1965, p. 102.
14. Fox, D. G.: An emperical study of the application of a horizontal uni-directional air-flow system for a hospital operating room. Thesis, Univ. of Minnesota, july 1967.

15. JAMES, K. W., JAMESON, B., KAY, H. E. M., LYNCH, J., NGAN, H.: Some practical aspects of intensive cytotoxic therapy. Lancet 1967 I, 1045.
16. KONING, J. DE, DOOREN, L. J., BEKKUM, D. W. VAN, ROOD, J. J. VAN, DICKE, K. A., RÁDL, J.: Transplantation of bone-marrow cells and fetal thymus in an infant with lymphopenic immunological deficiency. Lancet 1969 I, 1223.
17. LANDY, J. J.: Germfree techniques in patient care. IX. intern. Congress for microbiology. Moscow Pergamon Press (1966), p. 383.
18. LEVITAN, A. A., PERRY, S.: The use of an isolator system in cancer chemotherapy. Amer. J. Med. 44, 234 (1967).
19. — SCHULTE, F. L., STRONG, C. D., PERRY, S.: Bacteriologic surveillance of the patient isolator system. Arch. environm. Hlth 14, 837 (1967).
20. MCDADE, J. J., SABEL, F. L., AKERS, R. L., WALKER, R. J.: Microbiological studies on the performance of a laminar airflow biological cabinet. Appl. Microbiol. 16, 1086 (1968).
21. — WHITCOMB, J. G., RYPKA, E. W., WHITFIELD, W. J., FRANKLIN, C. M.: Microbiological studies conducted in a vertical laminar airflow surgery. J. Amer. med. Ass. 203, 125 (1968).
22. MEINDERSMA, T. E., WAAY, D. VAN DER: Observations on isolators for patients. Folia med. neerl. 11, 76 (1968).
23. MICHAELSEN, G. S., VESLEY, D., HALBERT, M. M.: Laminar flow studied as aid in care of low-resistance patients. Hospitals 41, 91 (1967).
24. RITTENBURY, M. S., HUME, D. M., HENCH, M. E.: "Pathogen-free" patient-care area. Conference Proc. Chicago 1962, p. 51.
25. ROELANTS, P., BOON, B., LHOEST, W.: Evaluation of a commercial air filter for removal of viruses from the air. Appl. Microbiol. 16, 1465 (1968).
26. RUCH, T. C., PATTON, H. D.: Physiology and biophysics. Philadelphia: Saunders Comp. 1965.
27. SCHNEIDER, M., SCHWARZENBERG, L., AMIEL, J. L., CATTAN, A., SCHLUMBERGER, J. R., HAYAT, M., VASSAL, F. DE, JASMIN, CL., ROSENFELD, CL., MATHÉ, G.: Pathogen-free isolation unit—three years' experience. Brit. med. J. 1969 I, 836.
28. SHADOMY, S., GINSBERG, M. K., LACONTE, M., ZEIGER, E.: Evaluations of a patient isolator system. Arch. environm. Hlth 11, 183, 191, 652 (1965).
29. STAAT, R. H., BEAKLEY, J. W.: Evaluation of laminar flow microbiological safety cabinets. Appl. Microbiol. 16, 1478 (1968).
30. TREXLER, P. C., REYNOLDS, L. I.: Flexible film apparatus for the rearing and use of germfree animals. Appl. Microbiol. 5, 406 (1957).
31. WAAY, D. VAN DER: The persistent absence of enterobacteriaceae from the intestinal flora of mice following antibiotic treatment. J. infect. Dis. 118, 32 (1968).
32. — ANDREAS, A. H.: Results obtained with the use of the laminar flow system. Prevention of contamination and cross-contamination tested with germ-free mice. Submitted for publication. Lab. Animal Care 1969.
33. WINSLOW, C. E. A., HERRINGTON, L. P.: Temperature and human life. Princeton 1949.
34. YATES, G., BODEY, G. P.: Laminar air for cancer patients. Contamination Control J. 1968, p. 20.

Monographs already Published